UNDERSTANDING HEALTH CARE BUDGETING

Allen G. Herkimer, Jr., Ed.D., FACHE, FHFMA
Associate Professor
Graduate Program in Health Administration
Southwest Texas State University
San Marcos, Texas

AN ASPEN PUBLICATION®
Aspen Publishers, Inc.
Rockville, Maryland
Royal Tunbridge Wells
1988

Library of Congress Cataloging-in-Publication Data

Herkimer, Allen G.
Understanding health care budgeting.

Bibliography: p.
Includes index.
1. Health facilities--Finance. I. Title.
RA971.3.H465   1988   362.1'1'0681   88-12602
ISBN: 0-87189-772-5

Editorial Services: Carolyn Ormes

Library of Congress Catalog Card Number: 88-12602
ISBN: 0-87189-772-5

Printed in the United States of America

1 2 3 4 5

To
health care managers I've known and
to those I've yet to meet

Table of Contents

Preface

The Third Wave economy will favor self-starters, doers, but it will also need creative dreamers in larger numbers than before. It will favor—and this is crucial—those who are future-oriented over those who live primarily in the past. And so on.

Alvin Toffler
Previews & Premises

Risk. Price. Cost. Productivity. These are the primary components managers must contend and work with today and in the health care economic environment of the future. Each component must be considered in terms of its futurity.

This is what budgeting is all about.

The state and federal governments have established regulatory commissions to "control" health care costs. The strategy is to control the amount of money third party payers have to pay to facilities; there is no attempt to control directly internal operating costs. The author of this book is committed to the view that only through effective internal management can health care facilities ever hope to successfully control operating costs.

To control health care costs and develop a successful budgetary control system, the key individual is the department manager. This person is in the best position to know how much a department's services are utilized and what its resources are. Accordingly, this person should be given the authority and responsibility for controlling the operating results of a specific responsibility center or department.

This book is intended to serve as a guide for department managers, supervisors, and nonaccountant health care managers of all levels in establishing their departmental budgetary control system and production management programs. Although the author encourages readers to utilize a microcomputer in developing the budget, the approach presented here can be manually applied. One of the advantages of using a microcomputer is that it affords the user the opportunity to make sensitivity and "what-if" testings.

The book emphasizes the need to measure quantifiably a health care department's services and/or product lines and to incorporate these data into a variable budgetary control system. The variable budget methodology, which is relatively new to the health care industry, offers the unique opportunity for managers to compensate for and to analyze volume variances. Using this methodology, management will be provided information with which to evaluate a department's productivity efficiency, as well as its financial performance.

This book provides the reader with the methodology to

- identify the production unit
- determine the cost of the production unit
- establish a selling price per production unit
- serve as a basis for evaluating operating performance in a quantitative as well as a financial mode

The health care organizations which will survive and grow in this new competitive health care environment will be enterprising, future- and risk-oriented, and capable of quickly adapting to the changes and needs of the marketplace. They will know their present and future product line costs and can price these products and/or services competitively and profitably. Budgeting is a tool which can assist these successful enterprising health care organizations. Quite simply, it's the Darwinian theory applied to health care finance and economics.

Allen G. Herkimer, Jr.
San Marcos, Texas
June, 1988

Acknowledgments

There are two groups to whom I express my heartfelt gratitude. The first group is composed of the many health care professionals and students whom I have had the good fortune and privilege to work and socialize with during my more than 30 years in the health care industry. These individuals contributed immeasurably to my knowledge of health care budgeting. They provided a forum for the constant exchange of ideas and concepts that has stimulated me to write this book.

The second group is composed of present-day health care managers—department managers, chief financial officers, budget directors, chief executive officers, and health administration students—who are no longer satisfied with the way it's always been done and instead are in search of a better way to manage health care institutions. These individuals are continually striving for excellence; they are the health care leaders of tomorrow. I have sincere faith in their desire and ability to help this nation's health care delivery system improve efficiency and productivity with a minimum of governmental intervention and control.

People form the core of our economic wealth; they are the means of production. In the Industrial Age, people aided machines; today, machines aid people.

Samuel E. Bleecher
The Futurist

Chapter 1

Health Care Budgeting

One of management's most widely used tools for the financial planning and control of a health care organization's operations is budgeting, and while it is not in itself a management tool, it becomes one through management action.[1]

The budget should be the result of a joint effort by the administration and the management team and their joint pledge to the governing body as to what the organization's operating plans for the future are. In essence, the budget serves as the organization's standard of operational expectations for the ensuing year(s), a standard by which its performance can be evaluated not only by the board but by management itself. The budget is a manifestation of management's knowledge, experience, and reasonable expectations expressed in quantitative and financial terms. The budget is truly the end result of applied humantology.

DEFINITION OF BUDGETING

Budgeting has been defined as the formulation of plans for a given future period in numerical terms. As such, budgets are statements of anticipated results expressed in financial terms (e.g., revenue and expense and capital budgets) or in nonfinancial terms (e.g., budgets of direct labor hours, materials, physical sales volume, or units of production). Financial budgets have sometimes been said to represent the ''dollarizing'' of plans.[2]

For our purposes, a budget will be defined as the systematic documentation of one or more carefully developed plans for all individually supervised activities, programs, or sections. These individually supervised cost centers, frequently referred to as responsibility centers, are coordinated into a departmental budget. Departmental budgets are further consolidated into a health care institution's master budget.[3]

Basically, budgeting is a planning and control device whose success can be measured in direct proportion to the attention given it by the individuals who are responsible for developing and administering the program—the humantology of budgeting.

The two planning and control models which are commonly used in health care budgeting are (1) strategic and (2) tactical. These models are designed to make financial planning and control an automatic process and to minimize crisis planning and management. They require health care managers to be constantly evaluating the present status of their institutions (both internal and external) with respect to future market needs.

STRATEGIC AND TACTICAL PLANNING

Strategic planning is usually conducted at the highest levels of an organization's management hierarchy (i.e., its governing boards and administration) at the time the organization's mission and goals are decided on and the strategies required to achieve these goals are identified. Through the strategic planning process, an organization's attention is directed to the future, thereby enabling it to adapt more readily to change and also to determine the direction in which the organization chooses to move.[4] It does this by continually evaluating the impact of change on the organization and its activities. The key to the process lies, first, in anticipating new conditions that promise to affect what the organization does or hopes to do in the future and, second, in then taking whatever actions are necessary to exploit these new conditions to the organization's own advantage and to the advantage of those whom it serves.[5]

Strategic planning does not deal with future decisions but with the futurity of today's decisions.[6] These decisions should ultimately be made by top management, but the planning process should not be their responsibility exclusively. They must be aware of and sensitive to the ideas, thoughts, and creativity that exist at the lower management level and be aware of and sensitive to the community's market needs and trends. However, they are obviously responsible for the final decisions, which will depend largely on their overall management philosophy.

It is critical to any successful strategic planning process that all those involved are constantly aware of the changing trends, the market needs, the technological advancements, and their implications for the institution so as to cope with and to operate within the changing environment.

Strategic planning is defined as the process of appraising the present operating environment, anticipating the future environment, establishing a specific set of goals (including the competitive position that the organization wants to achieve), and plotting a series of short-range tactical plans, preferably in one year incre-

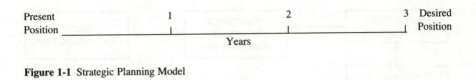

Figure 1-1 Strategic Planning Model

ments, which systematically route the organization toward its intended long-range position.

The strategic planning process can be equated with a series of photographs. The first picture depicts the position of the organization as it is. Another displays how management envisions the organization will look at some future time. Between these two are a series of photos showing progress from the first setting to the future target.

Using a three-year horizon, the strategic planning model, illustrated in Figure 1-1,

- appraises the organization's present position
- determines the organization's desired position
- describes the strategy by means of three tactical plans the organization is required to implement in order to achieve the desired position

Generally, tactical planning and control involve an integrated series of one-year tactical plans or operating budgets that are designed to assist the organization in achieving its strategic goals in a prudent and timely manner. The development of the operating (tactical) budget(s) of the organization is conducted during this planning and control process. Each annual budget is an incremental segment of the overall strategic plan. The tactical or budgetary planning process, illustrated in Figure 1-2, requires

1. establishing the organization's mission, goals, and objectives
2. identifying the budget's assumptions, variable standard rates and costs, acceptable performance standards, and other relevant guidelines
3. developing a capital expenditure plan
4. projecting a volume forecast
5. constructing a revenue and expense budget
6. forecasting the cash flow resulting from the preceding functions

The performance evaluation function of the budgetary planning and control model is the one function often ignored or ineffectively managed. The objective of the performance evaluation process is to compare the actual performance (i.e.,

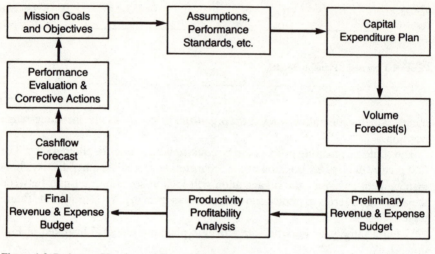

Figure 1-2 Budgetary Planning and Control Model

dollars and statistical volume and standards) to the budgeted amounts. Unacceptable performance variances must be promptly identified and corrective measures implemented in a timely and appropriate manner. The performance evaluation process, which utilizes the performance standards established in the planning process, comprises the following functions:

1. development of comparative management reports which display side by side the actual performance and the budgeted amounts on a monthly and year-to-date basis
2. variance analyses of *each* volume, revenue, and expense account
3. determination of whether *each* variance is favorable or unfavorable
4. identification and implementation of corrective measures to improve the unfavorable variances
5. re-evaluation and adjustment of the original performance standards, when appropriate

This budgetary planning and control model can be used, with minor variations, in either a strategic or a tactical mode. The basic difference would be that (1) the strategic planning process operates within a minimum of a three-year horizon and (2) the tactical planning approach is usually confined to a one-year horizon.

The tactical planning and control model which will be used throughout this book concentrates on preparing the department managers to be accountable for their departments or responsibility centers. Thus, the term *responsibility budgeting* will appear frequently. The hypothesis is that the department manager is in the most advantageous position to know what is needed to improve productivity and profitability in each revenue/cost center and to institute timely corrective measures and that therefore he or she should be held responsible for a specific cost/revenue center.

BENEFITS OF BUDGETING

There are numerous benefits to be derived from the budgeting process, but none of them can be realized unless there is total commitment at all levels of management. People, not computers, make the budget work.

Assuming that the commitment is present, some of the many benefits of a budgetary planning and control program are as follows:

- It places everyone on the management team.
- It helps to create cost awareness.
- It helps to measure individual and departmental productivity and profitability.
- It can produce savings and help to reduce waste.
- It helps to minimize the number of operational surprises, e.g., cash shortages, operating losses, etc.
- It provides all levels of management with a set of predetermined operating standards with which to evaluate operating performances.
- It serves as an excellent means of educating and developing managers.[7]

Finally, a properly planned and executed operational budget program frees top management so that it can concentrate on developing strategies for future institutional growth.

PREREQUISITES OF BUDGETING

The budget as a plan for the future must be based on an analysis of actual historical data, experience, or knowledge, which must be utilized separately or in combination to predict future operations and to aid management as it strives to reach a desired set of goals and objectives.

Again, the budget requires commitment from people, and this commitment must start right at the top with the governing board. The board has the fiduciary responsibility to preserve and maintain the institution's financial viability. Since financial viability is one of the primary purposes of budgeting, the first and foremost prerequisite is the board's total commitment to the budgetary program. After this has been achieved and management is in accord, other prerequisites for an effective budgetary control program are as follows:

1. an *organization structure*, with responsibility centers or departments identified and individual responsibility assigned
2. an accounting *chart of accounts* that parallels the organization chart and its responsibility centers or departments
3. an identified set of *departmental production units* that are easily recorded and audited and which are relevant to the type of work performed and to the amount of resources required to generate these production units
4. a *data collection system* that is designed to efficiently and, if possible, automatically collect related statistical and financial data on a concurrent and historical basis
5. a *management reporting system* that parallels the organization structure, the chart of accounts, and the budget
6. the identification of someone as the *budget director*, with responsibility for coordinating the budgetary process
7. the formation of a *budget committee*, with the budget director acting as chairperson; the budget committee is responsible for coordinating the budgetary process
8. a *budget calendar* that identifies developmental tasks, individual responsibilities, and timelines for the completion of each task
9. a *budget manual* that includes the uniform budget report forms and related instructions; the chart of accounts; the organization chart(s); the budget calendar; a list of budget committee members; the established institutional mission, goals, and objectives; the budgetary assumptions and operating performance standards identified by the board and/or top management; and other relevant information and forms

One piece of information that is helpful but not absolutely necessary to have, especially in the case of a new enterprise, is the previous year's actual financial and statistical data and the current year's data up to the date when the budgetary process begins. The current year's data are usually available through the first six to eight months of the year, and then they are annualized for the remainder of the year. Annualization of a partial year's data is discussed in Chapter 2.

ROLE OF THE GOVERNING BOARD

The institution's governing board assumes its responsibilities from the beginning of the budgeting process and remains involved throughout the program. As stated previously, its total commitment is absolutely essential, and when the commitment is made, the board, usually through its finance committee and in conjunction with administration, evaluates and updates the institution's mission. With its mission as a foundation, the finance committee and administration establish a set of goals and related quantitative objectives which spell out the desired operating results for the budget year. Together with some operating assumptions which reflect both the external and internal environments, these guidelines are transmitted to the chief financial officer, the budget director, and the institution's budget committee to serve as the criteria for developing the institutional budget on a departmental basis.

Upon completion of the institution's budget, it is presented to the board's finance committee for review and approval. It is not unusual to have the initial or preliminary budget rejected by the finance committee and returned to the budget committee for revision. When the budget is accepted by the finance committee, the committee recommends to the chairperson of the board that it be added to the next meeting's agenda (or to a special meeting's agenda) for review and approval.

Usually on a monthly basis, the board's finance committee receives budget reports of actual performance, budgetary expectations, and variance analyses and reviews them with management and the budget director; it then proceeds to make such recommendations as it believes necessary for assuring the achievement of the established budgetary goals and objectives. Once the recommendations for changes are made, it becomes the responsibility of management to implement the changes.

ROLE OF ADMINISTRATION

As far as the budgetary control program is concerned, there are generally two or three top administrative positions: the chief executive officer (CEO), the chief operating officer (COO), and the chief financial officer (CFO). The CEO, who is ultimately responsible for the execution of the board's policies, reports directly to the board and serves as the liaison between the board and the institution. In some health care institutions, the COO is responsible for the day-to-day operations of the institution, while the CEO may be more involved with the developmental and political functions, e.g., public relations, fund raising, marketing, planning, expansion, etc.

The CFO, who is ultimately responsible for the financial viability of the institution, usually reports directly to the CEO. The CFO is responsible for the collection, processing, reporting, and analysis of financial and statistical data; in some institutions the CFO may also serve as the budget director.

Many CFOs, recognizing the budget's importance as a management tool, have identified and assigned one individual to be the organization's budget director.

The budget director, who usually reports to the CFO, is responsible for the entire budgetary control program and may also serve as the chairperson of the budget committee.

BUDGET COMMITTEE AND ITS ROLE

The budget committee generally consists of a representative cross section of the major functional areas or divisions within the institution, with the designated budget director usually serving as the chairperson. Budget committees frequently include, among others, those who hold the following positions:

- *Director of Nursing.* This position is responsible for the major function of most health care institutions and also accounts for one of the largest, if not the largest, proportion of the institution's expenses and revenues.

- *Director of Human Resources.* This position is responsible for administering the institution's salary and wage program, including its hiring and firing policies. Since in most health care institutions salaries and wages constitute well over 50 percent of the organization's total operating expenses, the director of human resources is a valuable member of the budget committee.

- *Director of Materials Management.* This position represents the other half of the operating expense equation, the non-salary-and-wage expenses. The director of materials management provides knowledge of inflation trends; new market products; purchase and trade discounts; fixed asset requirements; and the requirements for receiving, storing, processing, pricing, and distributing the institution's operating supplies.

- *Director of Engineering and Plant Operations.* This position is responsible for the institution's building(s) and equipment, including repair and maintenance. The director of engineering and plant operations can provide a wealth of information about such things, as well as experience in new construction, remodeling, utilities efficiency, and other areas of concern.

- *Chief of Medical Staff.* This position represents the other half of the patient care equation, the medical staff. It is imperative that the physicians be represented in the budgetary planning and control process. They are not only the institution's major consumers, but they can be its best marketeers and salespersons. The medical staff, who are on or near the "cutting edge" of medical technology and therapy, can assist in identifying new procedures, treatments, and other related services which can benefit the institution and the community it serves.

- *Chief Executive Officer, Chief Operating Officer, and/or the Chief Financial Officer.* All three frequently serve as ex officio members of the budget committee. Their attendance at meetings and active interest in the budget committee's activities add credibility to the budget process and help to keep top management aware of the budget process, its direction, and the anticipated results.

ROLE OF THE DEPARTMENT MANAGER

Department managers clearly have one of the most critical functions in the budgetary planning and control process, for they serve as the link between the plans of administration and the performance of the institution's work force. If they fail to understand and accept the goals and objectives of the budget, they will never be able to communicate them to the individual employees and the desired results will not be achieved. Their total and active cooperation and commitment are essential for the budgetary program's success. Top management must also be totally committed to the program and must convey its support to every department manager.[8]

Department managers owe it to themselves and to the institution to be on the cutting edge of their specialties. These persons can best identify the areas where productivity can be improved and where services are needed to meet the demands of the marketplace and thus improve revenue. The department manager is strategically placed to recognize weaknesses in the program and to take appropriate corrective action in a timely manner. In many cases, the budgetary process assists administration in evaluating the performance of department managers. Administration should recognize that the organization's budget is going to be only as strong as its weakest manager. If a department manager is weak in financial expertise, it becomes administration's responsibility to guide, train, and develop this manager into becoming a knowledgeable, contributing member of the financial team.

BUDGET CALENDAR

The budget calendar is a budgetary planning and control instrument which serves as a performance guide. The budget calendar also

1. identifies, describes, and classifies the tasks required to complete the budgetary planning process
2. identifies the individual or group of individuals who are responsible for the successful and timely completion of the budgetary tasks
3. identifies the desired target date for the completion of the budgetary tasks

The budget calendar may be either displayed in a table of sequence format or in a Gantt chart format with related timelines, as illustrated in Exhibit 1-1.

Exhibit 1-1 Budget Calendar in Gantt Chart Format

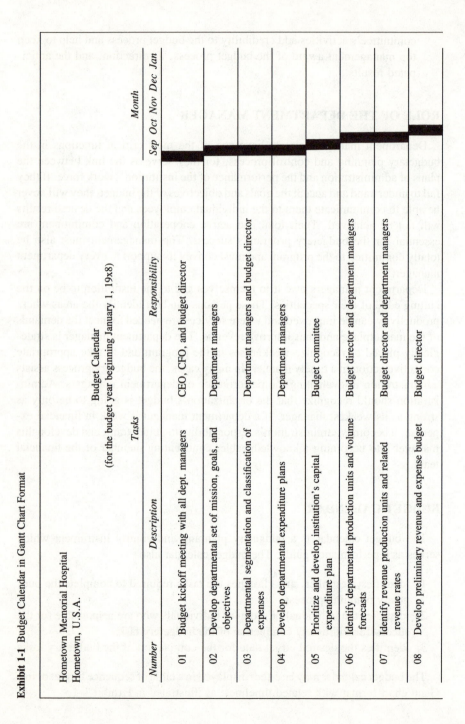

Hometown Memorial Hospital
Hometown, U.S.A.

Budget Calendar
(for the budget year beginning January 1, 19x8)

	Tasks		Month
Number	Description	Responsibility	Sep Oct Nov Dec Jan
01	Budget kickoff meeting with all dept. managers	CEO, CFO, and budget director	
02	Develop departmental set of mission, goals, and objectives	Department managers	
03	Departmental segmentation and classification of expenses	Department managers and budget director	
04	Develop departmental expenditure plans	Department managers	
05	Prioritize and develop institution's capital expenditure plan	Budget committee	
06	Identify departmental production units and volume forecasts	Budget director and department managers	
07	Identify revenue production units and related revenue rates	Budget director and department managers	
08	Develop preliminary revenue and expense budget	Budget director	

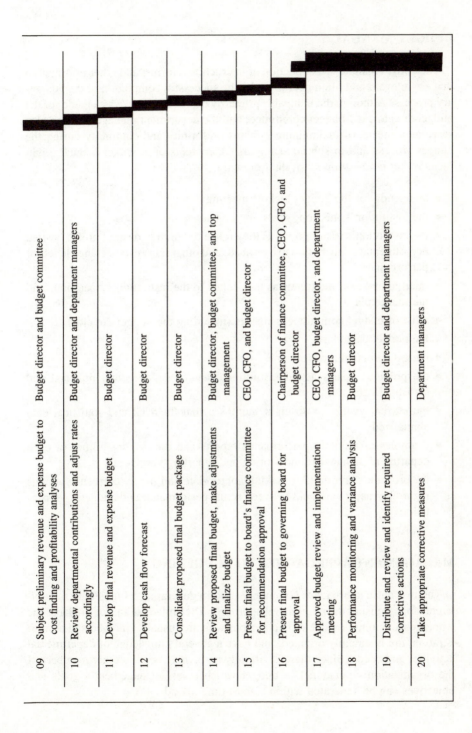

09	Subject preliminary revenue and expense budget to cost finding and profitability analyses	Budget director and budget committee
10	Review departmental contributions and adjust rates accordingly	Budget director and department managers
11	Develop final revenue and expense budget	Budget director
12	Develop cash flow forecast	Budget director
13	Consolidate proposed final budget package	Budget director
14	Review proposed final budget, make adjustments and finalize budget	Budget director, budget committee, and top management
15	Present final budget to board's finance committee for recommendation approval	CEO, CFO, and budget director
16	Present final budget to governing board for approval	Chairperson of finance committee, CEO, CFO, and budget director
17	Approved budget review and implementation meeting	CEO, CFO, budget director, and department managers
18	Performance monitoring and variance analysis	Budget director
19	Distribute and review and identify required corrective actions	Budget director and department managers
20	Take appropriate corrective measures	Department managers

BUDGET MANUAL

The budget manual is a collection of instructions, forms, and other information that are relevant and often necessary for the successful completion of the budgetary process. Although the manual is primarily designed to serve as a guide for the budget director, the budget committee, and the department managers, it can also serve as a means of maintaining systems uniformity and continuity during the budget process and in subsequent years. A contents of a budget manual might include, but not be limited to, the following:

- an agenda for the budget kickoff meeting
- the institution's mission, goals and objectives
- the institution's assumptions as they relate to volume, desired profit, desired departmental contribution to overhead, and other related expectancy levels of performance
- internal and external trends as they relate to the institution's operations and the marketplace
- a list of budget committee members (including the budget director)
- the budget calendar
- budget forms and instructions
- the previous year's actual institutional and/or departmental financial and statistical data
- the current year's six to eight months actual financial and statistical data annualized
- examples of monthly performance reports and the responsibilities of each department manager in monitoring and reporting variances
- the procedures required for taking appropriate and timely corrective actions regarding major variances between actual performance and budgetary expectations

MANAGEMENT APPROACHES TO BUDGETING

The two basic approaches commonly used in generating a budget are the unilateral approach and the multilateral approach. The unilateral approach places the whole responsibility on one or two persons who are (usually) members of administration, are financially oriented, and have a general knowledge of departmental activities and needs. Since there is virtually no involvement by other members of the organization's personnel, a budget which meets management's goals and objectives can be generated within a short time period.

The multilateral or participative approach can be a very cumbersome and slow process, because it requires that all individuals who are responsible for any revenue/cost center be involved in generating the budget as it applies to their areas. Although slow, this approach has its advantages. The department managers are being "sold" on the budget during their involvement in the mechanics of the budgeting process, and since they helped to generate the budget, they will make every effort to promote it and to operate within its established standards.

There are times when the unilateral approach may be necessary or especially desirable. If, for example, a budget program is urgently needed for a new service or acquisition, one person may be assigned the task of unilaterally generating a budget quickly. Another example is if an organization's management has never before had a budgetary control program. In such a situation, the faster a budget is developed and implemented, the better. Experience has shown, however, that the success of the program is more often assured if middle management participates from the beginning and that the multilateral approach is generally preferable.

TYPES OF BUDGETS

The type of budget selected for the institution will depend largely on the desired results. Traditionally, the fixed or static budget has been the most generally accepted. A fixed budget, however, has one major flaw: It cannot adjust its revenue and expenses to the volume variances which usually occur between the planned and the actual volume. A variable budget, on the other hand, accommodates and adjusts its variable revenues and expenses to the actual volume of activity, which is the main strength of the variable budget approach. This book is designed to present to the reader a methodology which can assist in the implementation of a variable budget program, but it is good to know all of the budget types available, some of which are described below.

The Fixed or Static Budget

This type of budget is developed and based on one volume of activity. Fixed budget methodologies generally do not require the separation of fixed and variable expenses, thus making it difficult to compare actual performance with the budgeted performance when the volume of activity differs.

The Target Budget

The target budget is developed in the same way as the fixed budget—it is generated by using a fixed volume of activity. However, the target budget requires expenses to be separated into either fixed or variable classifications. This segmentation of expenses provides the mechanics which are necessary for the development of (1) standard revenue rates per production units and (2) standard expense rates per production units for every variable salary and nonsalary expense item.

These standard rates, which are based upon a single targeted volume of activity, are incorporated into the variable budget methodology to adjust its "control budget" to the actual volume. Thus, the problem of explaining the differences which may be created by volume variances is eliminated.

The Variable Budget

This type of budget uses the standard variable rates generated in the target budget. By multiplying these rates by either their actual or budgeted daily, monthly, or annual volume, the total revenues and expenses for the accounting period can be generated. In the meantime, the segmented fixed salary and nonsalary expenses developed in the target budget remain constant, regardless of any changes in volume activity.

The Appropriation Budget

This type of budget may be classified as a systematic method for going into debt, because it is designed to be more of a "spending plan" than a managerial incentive or cost control device. The appropriation budget is most commonly used by governments and municipalities. The amounts of expenditures are usually fixed by some external body which appropriates funds for a specific department or division within the organization. Frequently, the total expenses of the budget serve as the basis by which the tax rate is computed. The primary weakness in this type of budget is that most managers of cost centers are encouraged to spend the total allotted expenses so that the next year's budget is not reduced accordingly. The basic incentive in many appropriation budget systems appears to be "spend it this year or lose it next year."

The Program Budget

The meaning of *program budget*, sometimes referred to as *project budget*, has not become standardized through general use. To some it suggests no more than a restructuring of budget exhibits by accumulating revenues and costs in more meaningful categories.[9] Basically, the program budget, which may include indirect as well as direct expenses, is designed to forecast the revenues and expenses of one specific project so as to assist management in monitoring the profitability of a new service. The program budget may cover a future period of one or more years, or until such time as the project is expected to become a profitable venture. Though the program budget is an effective management tool in forecasting and evaluating the cost/benefit of a single project, it should be considered only as a supplement to the institution's master budget plan.

Zero-Base Budgeting

This approach to budgeting is a relatively recent innovation in the budget control process. It was first implemented by Texas Instruments and subsequently popularized by former President Jimmy Carter, who, as governor, had used it in the state of Georgia and had planned to implement the process in the federal government.

The zero-base budgeting approach begins with the premise that no department or program should last forever unless it can justify its existence. There are two basic steps required in the methodology: (1) development of decision packages and (2) ranking and prioritizing of decision packages. Each decision package identifies the project, department, or unit and includes its mission, goals, objectives, revenues, expenses, and its benefits to the entire organization.

Once decision packages are developed and ranked, management can allocate resources accordingly, funding the most important decision packages whether they are current or new. The final budget is produced by taking packages that are approved for funding, sorting them into their appropriate budget units, and adding the revenues and costs identified in each package to produce the organization's total budget.[10]

Zero-base budgeting can be a time-consuming process, but it can also be valuable for any floundering health care organization which is trying to recover its overall profitability.

THE BUDGET PROCESS

Budget methodology is discussed in detail throughout this book, but it is helpful at this point to get an overview of the major steps required to develop a health care variable budget program, which are as follows.

Step 1. At the budget kickoff meeting of department managers, the initial introduction of the budgetary planning and control program is presented by the CEO or the COO together with the CFO and the designated budget director. During this meeting, the institution's mission, goals, objectives, and some basic assumptions (e.g., inflation rate, desired macro volume activity, anticipated wage adjustment, etc.) for the budget year are presented and reviewed by the CEO or COO. This presentation affords an opportunity to clarify the objectives established by the institution's governing board, to demonstrate top management's support of the program, and to encourage total support by the department managers.

During the kickoff meeting, the budget manual, budget calendar, historical and current financial and statistical data, and any other relevant information are circulated among all department managers and gone over by either the CFO or the budget director.

Step 2. Each department manager is required to establish and document a departmental mission and departmental goals and objectives; these must be compatible with the institution's designated mission, goals, and objectives.

Step 3. Each department manager is required to negotiate with the budget director the segmentation of the department's expenses as either fixed or variable, and together they develop standard rates for each variable expense item.

Step 4. Department managers are required to generate a three-year capital expenditure plan and submit it to the budget director.

Step 5. The budget committee reviews all departmental capital expenditure plans and generates and approves an acquisition schedule for the institution. Department managers are notified of the committee's decisions and subsequently incorporate the related revenues and expenses into their departmental budgets.

Step 6. Each department manager, in conjunction with the budget director, identifies the appropriate departmental production unit(s), either macro or micro, and develops the department's monthly volume forecast.

Step 7. Each department manager, in conjunction with the budget director, identifies each service or product generated for sale by the department and registers the current price as the basis for projecting the preliminary revenue budget. Note: The preliminary revenue budget is usually based on the current pricing structure. If, after reducing the budgeted expenses to the minimum the desired operating profit is not projected, then and only then should prices be increased.

Step 8. The budget director collects all departmental budgets and generates the preliminary budget.

Step 9. The budget director subjects the preliminary budget to the cost finding process in order to identify any department which is not generating its desired contribution to the institution and to analyze why.

Step 10. The budget director, in conjunction with the appropriate department manager(s), reviews all departmental budgets which are not generating the desired institutional contribution. During this process, it is important that activity or productivity volumes be confirmed and expenses be minimized in order to keep a competitive edge. Only as a last resort should prices be increased.

Step 11. After all departmental budgets have been adjusted so as to achieve the desired departmental contributions and institutional operating results, the budget director generates a final institutional "master" operating budget.

Step 12. Using the institution's final master operating budget and capital expenditure plan, the budget director develops a monthly cash forecast. If the desired cash position is not projected, the budget director and the budget committee make recommendations (or ''budget balancers'') to top management. Budget balancers can be incorporated in the final master budget or submitted as an addendum to the preliminary budget for review and approval by the finance committee.

Step 13. The budget director consolidates and ''packages'' the institution's master budget documentation, which might include, but need not be limited to, the following:

- an executive summary
- the mission, goals, and objectives
- a description of assumptions
- a capital expenditure plan
- volume forecasts
- a comparative revenue and expense summary
- a cash flow forecast
- an appendix consisting of supporting documents and departmental budgets

Step 14. The budget committee and administration review the final master budget package and make appropriate additions or deletions, if needed.

Step 15. The final master budget package is submitted to the finance committee of the governing board for its approval. Note: Since approval is not always obtained during the initial budget presentation, time must be allotted for revisions and subsequent submissions to the finance committee.

Step 16. After approving the final budget, the finance committee presents it to the governing board and recommends its acceptance. The budget, after board approval, is ready for presentation to the institution's department managers.

Step 17. The board-approved budget program is distributed to all department managers at a budget implementation meeting similar to the budget kickoff meeting (Step 1). During this meeting, which is usually moderated by the CEO, the final master budget package is reviewed and officially prepared for implementation.

Step 18. After the organization has been operating for a short period, usually one month, the actual performance is compared to a ''control'' budget which has been adjusted to the actual volume of activity. During this step, revenue and expense performance analyses and variance ratios (i.e., efficiency, usage, and rates) are computed to identify favorable and unfavorable deviations from the planned achievements.

Step 19. The complete results of the comparative performance analysis computed in Step 18 are circulated and the budget director individually reviews them with each department manager. Each department manager is required to identify the causes for the significant variances (usually those over 5 percent) and to determine what appropriate corrective actions are required to assure that the department's designated contribution to the institution is attained. Note: It is important that both the favorable and the unfavorable variances be examined in order to adjust the budget forecasting procedure.

Step 20. While some corrective actions may be implemented without administrative approval, other changes may require it. Most important is that these corrective actions be implemented efficiently and in a timely manner.

The budget methodology illustrated in Figure 1-2 and described above should be considered only as a model from which a health care institution can develop its own budgetary planning and control program. Of primary importance is that successful budgeting cannot be implemented without the cooperation and participation of the department managers; they hold the key to any effective budgetary planning and control program.

NOTES

1. California Hospital Association and the California chapters of the Healthcare Financial Management Association, *CHA/HFMA Budgeting Manual*, 2d ed. (Sacramento: California Hospital Association, 1977), 3.

2. Harold Koontz, Cyril O'Donnell, and Heinz Weihrich, *Management*, 8th ed. (New York: McGraw-Hill, 1984), 571.

3. Allen G. Herkimer, Jr., *Understanding Hospital Financial Management*, 2d ed. (Rockville, Md.: Aspen, 1986), 144.

4. Joseph P. Peters, *Strategic Planning for Hospitals* (Chicago: American Hospital Association, 1979), 13.

5. Ibid.

6. Peter Drucker, "Long-Range Planning: Challenge to Management Science," *Management Science* 5 (1969): 17.

7. Allen G. Herkimer, Jr., *Concepts in Hospital Financial Management*, 2d ed., (San Marcos, Tex.: Alfa Management Services, 1973), 79–80.

8. Ibid., 94–95.

9. Herkimer, *Understanding Hospital Financial Management*, 147–56.

10. Ibid.

Budget Foundation and Guidelines

2

A clearly written, definitive budgetary planning and control plan is critical for the steady development and growth of any health care organization. Budgetary planning and control has been defined in many ways. One writer considers it to be an orderly process for setting organizational direction or preparing for change and coping with the uncertainty by formulating future courses of action.[1] Another views planning as "deciding what to do and how to do it before action is required,"[2] while yet another considers planning to be anticipating the future, which implies contending with environments.[3]

Incorporating these attributes, another author defines budgetary planning and control as anticipating the future, assessing present conditions, and making decisions concerning organizational direction, programs, and resource deployment.[4] This process results in answers to questions of what to do and when, where, how, and why.[5]

The basic budget foundation required to establish an effective budgetary planning and control program comprises the following:

1. Statement of mission
2. Statement of goals
3. Statement of objectives

Collectively, these three statements serve as the guidelines for developing an institutional and departmental budgetary planning and control program.

MISSION STATEMENT

The mission statement of an organization serves as the fundamental guideline for the budgeting process. This document states the main purpose(s) of the institution.

23

An organization may sometimes have a social purpose coupled with a business purpose. For example, a hospital or clinic may be dedicated to furnishing ambulatory health care services to the residents of Hometown, U.S.A.; it is also committed to returning a profit to its investors. While generating a profit is an absolute necessity for a growing business, the basic method used to achieve this profit is usually identified as the institution's mission.

The mission statement is supported by a comprehensive statement of goals and objectives. The goals of an organization are more specific than the mission. Each goal, in turn, is supported by a set of objectives, which are even more specific. Descriptions of objectives spell out exactly what is to be accomplished and within what timeframe.

These three steering mechanisms can be equated to an umbrella (see Figure 2-1). The mission, serving as the handle and staff of the umbrella, is the primary reason for the organization's existence. The goals, represented by the ribs or stays, support and complement the institution's mission. The umbrella covering or fabric represents the assortment of institutional and departmental objectives designed as the strategies to be used for the fulfillment of the organization's mission.

The mission statement is usually restricted to one or two concise paragraphs identifying the main purpose of the organization, including the services or products which provide its reason for existing. For instance, the mission statement of Hometown Memorial Hospital is as follows:

> To serve efficiently and effectively as the central medical center of Hometown, U.S.A., by rendering quality health care services at reason-

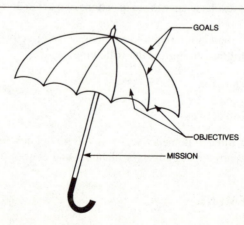

Figure 2-1 The Relationship between an Organization's Mission, Goals, and Objectives

able costs to the residents of Hometown, including, but not limited to, acute care, emergency services, home health care, an ambulatory clinic, health education, and other identified market needs.

This mission statement serves as the primary guideline for the individual department managers as they develop their individual departmental mission statements. For example, the mission statement of the laboratory department of Hometown Memorial Hospital might be as follows:

To effectively and efficiently render quality laboratory services to Hometown Memorial Hospital's inpatients and outpatients; to be continually aware of new laboratory-related health care needs in the hospital's marketplace; to constantly review, assess, and acquire appropriate technology; and to continually strive to improve the department's quality of service and its productivity.

It is vital that the organizational and departmental mission statements complement each other. Again, the facility's mission, as well as its goals and objectives, serves as the foundation supporting and directing its various departments toward well-defined ends.

Defining the purpose of the health care institution can be difficult, painful, and sometimes risky, but it is always necessary. It alone enables the organization to develop a set of goals and objectives, to develop strategies, to concentrate its resources, and to go to work. It alone enables the enterprise to be managed for performance and results.[6]

GOALS AND OBJECTIVES

The terms *goal* and *objective* are often confused and used interchangeably. The following should clarify how these terms are used in this text.

A goal is an expected result of using a specific strategy and a designated amount of resources. The statement of a goal describes what the general output (result) is intended to be when certain inputs (resources) are utilized by a system. For example, a goal for a patient business service department might be to reduce the number of days average daily revenue uncollected.

One or more objectives, usually described in quantitative terms and through projected timelines, are usually associated with a goal. They are more specific targets that assist in achieving the goal. The following is an example of a set of related goals and objectives for the patient business services department (see also Exhibit 2-1).

Exhibit 2-1 Statement of Goals and Objectives

Hometown Memorial Hospital
Hometown, U.S.A.   page 1 of 1

Goals and Objectives
for 1 Year Ending December 31, 19x2

Check One: ___ Strategic   _X_ Tactical

Department: _Patient Business Services_   Date: _September 15, 19x1_

Department Manager: _Gil Stevens_

Instructions: First, list and describe your department's strategic goals and objectives, giving their costs and anticipated completion dates; sequentially number them with an "S" prefix, e.g., S-1, S-2, etc. Second, list and describe the tactical goals and relevant information, numbering them with a "T" prefix, T1.1, T1.2, T1.3, etc.

Goals		Objectives and Estimated Cost	
Number	Description	Description and Cost	Date
S-1	to reduce the number of average days revenue uncollected	T1.1 to reduce the total number of days revenue uncollected by ten (10) days or one (1) million dollars, whichever is the greatest amount T1.2 to not increase the existing staff T1.3 to incur no additional expenses; to systematically increase productivity	

- Goal 1.0: to reduce the number of days average daily revenue uncollected
- Objective 1.1: to reduce the number of days of average daily revenue uncollected by ten days or one million dollars, whichever is greater

To summarize, the mission, goals, and objectives of an institution represent the hierarchy of management's desired results. The mission statement identifies the desired direction in which the organization is expected to go. The goals are the generally desired results, while the objectives quantitatively support each related goal. Objectives, while they must always relate to a specific goal, need not be restricted in number. What is important is that objectives specify the expected results for each related goal and when they are to be achieved. In essence, the objectives serve as the strategies to be used to achieve the goal. This facilitates the performance evaluation process and helps to identify performance variances.

BUDGET ASSUMPTIONS

The final (or master) budget comprises a series of detailed plans which are closely coordinated and integrated.[7] In order to assure that all departmental budgets in the organization are developed uniformly, administration and the budget committee assemble a list of assumptions which they believe should be incorporated in each department's forecast. These basic assumptions serve as guidelines for the department managers when they develop the departmental budgets and they may be incorporated in all or some of the departmental budgets, as appropriate.

Some examples of institutional assumptions are as follows:

- The inflation rate shall be calculated at five and one-half (5½%) percent.
- Inpatient days are anticipated to decrease three (3%) percent over the previous year.
- Outpatient visits are expected to increase twenty-five (25%) percent over the previous year.
- Department managers are expected to reduce their total departmental expenses by ten (10%) percent of the present operating level.
- Salary increases, which may be implemented on an employee's hiring date anniversary, may not exceed four (4%) percent.

Such institutional assumptions are then consolidated with each department's own list of assumptions and incorporated in its departmental budget. As the department manager develops the budget, it is frequently necessary to document additional assumptions related to the specific departmental budget. For example, the nursing department may decide to staff the nursing floor with a specific core or fixed staff of

1	Head registered nurse
3	Registered nurses
3	Licensed practical nurses
6	Nurse aides and/or orderlies
13	Total core staff

This staff will deliver 5.0 nursing hours per patient day; when the staffing ratio declines to 4.5 nursing hours per patient day, additional nursing staff may be hired from the registry.

It is imperative that whatever assumptions the department manager incorporates in the budget be documented. The documentation of assumptions can serve the department manager or budget director as a ''memory bank'' during the defense of the budget.

PRODUCTION UNITS

The selection of a department's most appropriate production unit (or units) is possibly the most critical decision a department manager has to make in the budgetary planning and control process. When any production unit is identified, the department manager has made a long-term commitment to use the unit for the following purposes:

1. to measure and evaluate the department's productivity
2. to measure and evaluate a departmental employee's productivity
3. to serve as the basis for computing the cost of the department's product
4. to serve as the basis for computing the selling price of the department's product
5. to serve as the basis for forecasting what the department expects to produce during the budget year
6. to serve as the basis for computing employee and/or machine production standards
7. to serve as the basis for determining staffing requirements

These are only a few of the many ways a department's production unit (or units) may be used in the budgetary planning and control process.

For its application in the health care budgetary planning and control program, a production unit is defined as the result (or output) of a system's use of resources over a specific period of time (see Figure 2-2).

Production units are usually measured by two basic methods. One, the macro method, identifies what is produced (e.g., patient days, outpatient visits, laboratory tests, radiology exams, etc.), but it does not try to establish what relationship between the amounts of any two resources is required to generate the macro production unit.

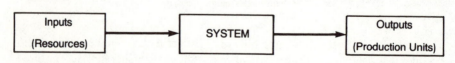

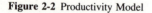

Figure 2-2 Productivity Model

Another type of production unit is the micro or relative value unit (RVU). This is more meaningful, because the micro system establishes a method with which to measure the amount of resources required to generate the production unit and consequently establishes a quantitative relationship between two outputs.

Finally, since a production unit identifies what each department is producing, it serves as the basis for projecting a department's volume of activity. It is, therefore, imperative that the selection of any production unit (or units) accurately reflects the department's outputs. The selection and uses of production units are discussed in greater detail in Chapters 3 and 5.

EXPENSE SEGMENTATION AND CLASSIFICATION

After the production units have been identified, the next task for each department manager, in cooperation with the budget director, is to segment and classify the department's direct operating expenses.

Direct expenses are the costs which are directly related to the performance of each department's assigned function (e.g., housekeeping, laundry, nursing, laboratory, etc.). All of the direct expenses can usually be controlled by the department manager and are therefore the only expenses which should be included in the identified departmental budgets.

One of the unique features of the variable budget process is that it requires all departmental expense items included in the chart of accounts to be segmented and classified as either a fixed or a variable expense (see Exhibit 2-2).

Regardless of the volume of work output, departmental fixed expense items tend to remain constant over a relevant period of time (see Figure 2-3). Insurance, depreciation, and rent are excellent examples of a department's fixed non-salary-and-wage costs. The salary of the department manager is a fixed salary and wage expense item.[8]

Departmental variable expense items tend to vary or change in direct relationship to the volume of units produced over a relevant period of time (see Figure 2-4). Food, x-ray films, drugs, and medical and surgical supplies are examples of variable non-salary-and-wage expense items. Nurse staffing and the resultant costs, which tend to require adjustments according to the patient census, are examples of departmental variable salary and wage expenses.[9] The composite of these departmental expense behaviors is illustrated in Figure 2-5.

Another expense classification which can be used in the variable budget process is the step-variable expense. Step-variable expenses are probably the most confusing kind of expense, because they are a combination of variable and fixed components. They tend to remain constant over a relevant range of activity and then change abruptly at intervals (see Figure 2-6). For example, regardless of the patient census, a nursing floor might have an established "core staff" of nursing

Exhibit 2-2 Segmentation of Revenue and Expenses

Hometown Memorial Hospital
Hometown, U.S.A.

Segmentation of Department Revenue and Expenses by Behavior

Department: Medical and Surgical Routine Nursing

Account Number	Account Description	Fixed Expenses	Variable Expenses
	Revenue		
3541.01	Private, 1-bed nursing services		X
3541.02	2-bed nursing services		X
3541.03	4-bed nursing services		X
	Deductions from Gross Revenue		
4541.01	Medicare allowances		X
4541.02	Medicaid allowances		X
4541.03	Blue Cross allowances		X
4541.04	Other contractual allowances		X
4541.05	Free work & charity		X
4541.10	Bad debts, less recoveries		X
	Salaries and Wages		
5541.01	Management & Supervision	X	
5541.03	Core registered nurses	X	
5541.04	Core licensed practical nurses	X	
5541.05	Core nurse aides & orderlies	X	
5541.08	P.R.N. nursing staff		X
5541.09	Ward clerks & other clerical	X	
5541.10	Employee benefits	X	
	Non-Salary-and-Wage Expenses		
6541.15	Office supplies		X
6541.19	Medical & surgical supplies		X
6541.21	Dues & subscriptions	X	
6541.22	Pharmaceuticals		X
6541.25	Depreciation	X	
6541.26	Insurance	X	
6541.27	Equipment leases	X	
6541.28	Training programs and conferences	X	
6541.29	Educational travel expenses	X	
6541.30	Recruitment fees & expenses	X	
6541.35	Registry fees		X
6541.50	Other operating expenses		X

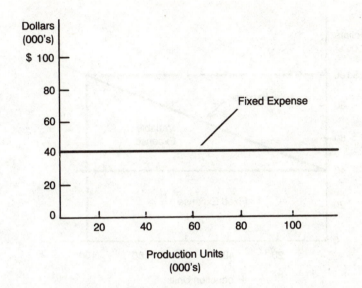

Figure 2-3 Departmental Fixed Expenses

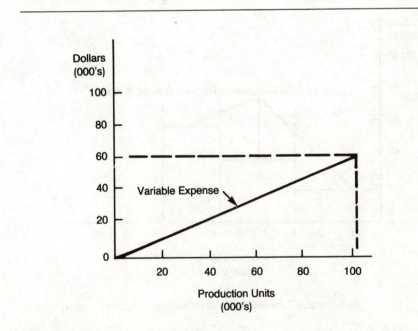

Figure 2-4 Departmental Variable Expenses

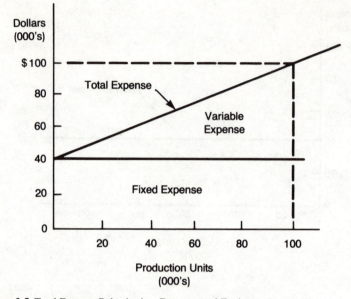

Figure 2-5 Total Expense Behavior in a Departmental Environment

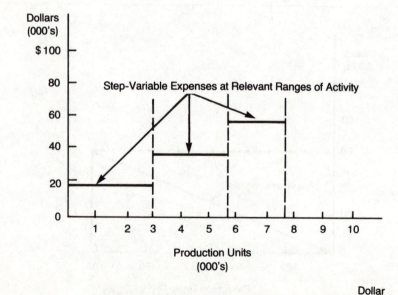

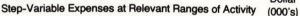

Step-Variable Expenses at Relevant Ranges of Activity   Dollar (000's)

Figure 2-6 Departmental Step-Variable Expenses at Relevant Ranges of Activity

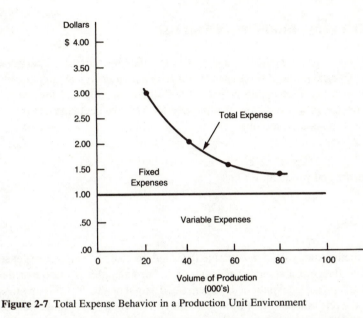

Figure 2-7 Total Expense Behavior in a Production Unit Environment

personnel. The expenses for this group are classified as ''fixed.'' But if the patient census exceeds its predicted level, the nursing staff may have to be increased; the expenses would then be classified as step-variable.

We have discussed expense behavior as it is defined and illustrated in a departmental environment, but it is important to know that expense behavior reacts almost conversely when it is measured within production unit surroundings. For example, the fixed expense component of the total cost of a production unit becomes less and less as the volume that is produced increases, while the variable expense component tends to remain the same over a relevant range of activity (see Figure 2-7 and Table 2-1).

Table 2-1 Comparative Analysis of Total Departmental and Total Production Unit Expenses Based on Volume of Activity

	Volume of Production Units					
	20,000		*40,000*		*80,000*	
Description	*Department Expense*	*Unit Cost*	*Department Expense*	*Unit Cost*	*Department Expense*	*Unit Cost*
Variable expenses	$20,000	$1.00	$40,000	$1.00	$ 60,000	$1.00
Fixed expenses	40,000	2.00	40,000	1.00	40,000	.50
Total expenses	$60,000	$3.00	$80,000	$2.00	$100,000	$1.50

STANDARD RATES: DEFINITION AND USE

A standard rate represents the average cost or revenue of a variable expense or revenue item. For example, if the expenses for medical and surgical supplies for the routine nursing service department total $324,870 annually and the annual patient days for the relevant period of time total 54,326, the standard rate (cost) would be $5.98, computed as follows:

$$\frac{\text{Total department variable expenses}}{\text{Total departmental production units}} = \text{standard rate (cost)}$$

or

$$\frac{\$324,870}{54,326} = \$5.98$$

The same methodology used to compute the standard cost of a variable expense item is used to develop a standard revenue rate. For example, assume that the 54,326 medical and surgical patient days generated a total of $10,593,570 in gross charges. For the relevant period of time, the standard revenue rate would be $195, computed as follows:

$$\frac{\text{Total annual gross revenue (charges)}}{\text{Total annual patient days}} = \text{standard revenue rate}$$

or

$$\frac{\$10,593,570}{54,326} = \$195$$

In the variable budget process each revenue and expense item requires an assigned standard rate, which is then multiplied by the volume of activity for a specific period of time. For example, the total monthly gross revenue and medical and surgical supply expenses for the year 19x2 would be computed as illustrated in Table 2-2.

HISTORICAL DATA: USE AND ANNUALIZATION

As a general rule, most budget projections are based on a health care institution's own historical financial and statistical information. These data represent the most reliable and relevant "hard data" from which to identify trends in activity, revenue, expenses, and other key indices. When historical information is not available, industrial revenue, expense, staffing, and production standards may be

Table 2-2 Medical and Surgical Routine Service Nursing Department Computation of Monthly Gross Revenue and Medical and Surgical Supply Expenses Using Standard Rates for the Year Ending December 31, 19x5

Month	Patient Days	Gross Revenue		Medical and Surgical Expenses	
		Standard	*Total*	*Standard*	*Total*
January	4,800	$195.00	$ 936,000	$5.98	$28,704
February	4,291	195.00	836,745	5.98	25,660
March	4,530	195.00	883,350	5.98	27,089
April	4,609	195.00	898,755	5.98	27,562
May	4,546	195.00	886,470	5.98	27,185
June	4,291	195.00	836,745	5.98	25,660
July	4,132	195.00	805,740	5.98	24,709
August	4,390	195.00	856,050	5.98	26,252
September	4,609	195.00	898,755	5.98	27,562
October	4,927	195.00	960,756	5.98	29,463
November	4,751	195.00	926,445	5.98	28,412
December	4,450	195.00	867,750	5.98	26,612
Total	54,326		$10,593,570		$324,870

substituted, such as those generated by the American Hospital Association and its Hospital Administrative Services' Montitrend and those generated by the Healthcare Financial Management Association's Financial Analysis Service (FAS). Regardless of which base data are used, they must be uniform and relevant to the organization and to the budget being developed.

Two historical data bases—the one for the previous year and the one for the current year—are usually used to project next year's budget.

Under most circumstances, the budget preparation process starts after 6 or 8 months into the current year. Since both data bases must be relevant, the current year's partial data must be ''annualized'' to be relevant to the previous year's data. Annualization is the process by which the actual statistical and financial data (e.g., 6 months data) are projected, as an estimate, for a period of 12 months. The annualization process makes an institution's partial year data relevant to the complete 12 months actual data from the previous year.

Using the data in Table 2-3 and knowing that the current year's 6 months data are from the period January 1 through June 30, we can assume that the current year's data represent 181 calendar days and that 184 calendar days need to be estimated and added so as to arrive at an annualized total. Further assuming that there will be no significant changes in operations for the remaining 6 months, the annualization process may be computed as illustrated in Table 2-4.

Table 2-3 Comparative Summary Analysis of Patient Days, Revenue, and Expenses for the Fiscal Year Ending December 31, 19x5 and the Six-Month Period Ending June 30, 19x6

	Actual		Estimate
	12 Months 19x1 Previous Year	6 Months 19x2 Current Year	12 Months 19x2 Current Year
Patient days	54,326	27,242	NA
Net revenue	$9,366,950	$4,663,475	NA
Net expense	8,124,780	4,162,390	NA
Net profit	$1,242,170	$ 501,085	NA

Table 2-4 Computation of the Annualization of Patient Days, Revenue, and Expenses for the Current Fiscal Year Ending December 31, 19x5 and Based on the Six Months Actual Data Ending June 30, 19x6

Description	Patient Days	Net Revenue	Net Expense
Six months actual	27,242	$4,663,475	$4,162,390
Number of calendar days in period	181	181	181
Average per calendar day	150.5	$ 25,765	$ 22,996
Number of days to be projected	365	365	365
Current year's six months data annualized total	54,932	$9,404,225	$8,393,540

The 12 months estimate of the current year's data needed to complete the comparative analysis in Table 2-3 are as follows:

Summary of Annualized Six-Month Data
for Fiscal Year Ending December 31, 19x6

Patient days	54,932
Net revenue	$9,404,225
Net expense	8,393,540
Net profit	$1,010,685

This methodology, one of many approaches to annualization, computes an average calendar day's activity and then projects the estimated annual total as the product of the average value multiplied by the number of calendar days in the year (i.e., 365 days or, in the case of a leap year, 366 days).

Uniformity is the key word in the accumulation and projection of a health care organization's historical data. Lack of uniformity in defining an institution's terms (e.g., production units) may lead to mistaken or inequitable interpretations, comparisons, and judgments. Financial and statistical reports are meaningful only when the data are accumulated and analyzed consistently and uniformly. To assure continuity of data, terms which are commonly used throughout the institution (e.g., pounds of laundry, operating room minutes, etc.) should be included in the budget manual.[10]

Uniform historical data can assist health care managers in identifying organizational and departmental trends. It may be beneficial to compare operating results of other health care organizations, but if the data are not relevant, the comparison may be misleading and confusing. What is important is that an organization's departmental internal operating results be routinely compared to and analyzed with those projected in the budget.

Occasionally, these historical data need to be supplemented with other known facts about the future, for example, the competition's prices, the competition's new services, the market's wage scale, local demographic trends, increases in key expense items such as insurance, fuel, utilities, etc. Each known fact which may affect the organization's future operations must be evaluated and the relevant information must be incorporated in the budget.[11]

OTHER RELEVANT BUDGET CONSIDERATIONS

Other relevant considerations which must be evaluated during the budget development process can be divided into two major areas: (1) the internal environment and (2) the external environment.

The internal environment must be examined from a corporate structure standpoint in order to determine if the organization is designed so as to be flexible enough to cope with competition, to penetrate markets with new products or services, and to raise sufficient capital to support existing and new enterprises. It is also important to consider, to evaluate, and perhaps to invest in opportunities within the taxable environment, yet still be able to retain the advantages of a nontaxable entity's corporate structure (e.g., tax-free bonds, grants, donations, etc.).

The external environment primarily comprises four sections: (1) competition, (2) legislation, (3) technology, and (4) systems.

Competition

Critical to an organization's survival is that it have a thorough knowledge of its competition. Competition can come from an organization which operates basically as the same type of structure (e.g., hospital versus hospital) or from a dissimilar organization (e.g., hospital versus medical group). Regardless of the source, a health care organization has only a few alternatives if it wants to outlast its competitors:

- It can give up wherever the competition appears too strong.
- It can fight its competition and try to secure the desired market share.
- It can cooperate, even if it means accepting a reduced share of the market, but at less cost in effort.[12]

Legislation

The federal and state governments, through their agencies, are the major third party payers of health care services, and they tend to influence most of the criteria, methods, and systems used by many of the other third party payers. As a consequence, the health care providers usually supply only the type of care or kinds of services these payers will cover. It becomes imperative, therefore, that health care managers be constantly aware of proposed and enacted laws, both federal and state (including the laws of states other than their own). It is not unusual for one state's successful experiment or specific legislation to be enacted and implemented in others, and every change affects the financial status of an institution.

Technical

In today's rapidly changing technological environment, physicians often demand the newest items in capital equipment. These sizeable investments must be subjected to a thorough cost-benefit analysis in order to evaluate the relevant potential benefit or loss to the institution and to its service area.

Systems

Health care managers have, through the years, developed alternative delivery systems (e.g.. urgent care, surgi-centers, home health care, etc.) to care for their patients more economically and to recapture lost revenues. A constant in the dynamics of health care delivery appears to be the trend away from inpatient acute care and toward preventive and ambulatory services. An organization's health care delivery system must be continually evaluated and adjusted so as to constantly meet market needs. The zero-base budgeting approach may be effectively used to evaluate and prioritize a health care organization's departments and services.

FORMAT OF BASIC DEPARTMENTAL BUDGET SPREADSHEET

The departmental variable budgeting methodology presented in this book is designed so that it may be generated in a manual mode or in a microcomputer system. Using the chart of accounts of Hometown Memorial Hospital's medical and surgical routine nursing services department (see Exhibit 2-2), the basic departmental budget, as formatted in Exhibit 2-3, has the following as its key information factors:

1. *File Name.* When computer application is used, the file name identifies the program designed for a specific department.
2. *Name of Health Care Organization.* To assure positive identification, the primary name of the health care organization should always be placed near the top of each departmental budget spreadsheet.
3. *Name of Department or Responsibility Center.* To assure proper recognition, the name of the department or responsibility center should be placed below the name of the organization.
4. *Length of Budget Period.* Since budget periods may vary in length of time and in starting and ending time, the length of budget time is usually placed near the top of the budget spreadsheet.
5. *Chart of Account Identifying Account Number.* The chart of account item number is used in the budget spreadsheet for positive identification of the related account item.
6. *Chart of Account Item Description.* The account description facilitates identification of the related account.
7. *Segmentation of Expenses.* To facilitate processing and account management, expense items are segmented as follows:

   • fixed salary and wages
   • fixed non-salary-and-wage expenses
   • variable salary and wages
   • variable non-salary-and-wage expenses

8. *Identification of Production Units.* A department may have more than one production unit. It is essential that all related production units be identified in order to assure continuity and understanding.
9. *Segmented Time Periods.* Budget time periods are usually segmented by month. Operating budget periods must correlate with the same time periods as those in the cash forecast statement.
10. *Distribution of Volume Production.* Production units are usually distributed on a monthly basis. These units represent the volume of work

Exhibit 2-3 Departmental Variable Budget

Hometown Memorial Hospital
Hometown, U.S.A.

Departmental Variable Budget
For Year Ending December 31, 19x3

Department: Medical and Surgical Routine Nursing

Account Number	Description	Standard Rate	January	February	March	April	May	June	July	August	September	October	November	December	Total
	Volume:														
	1-bed patient days														
	2-bed patient days														
	4-bed patient days														
	Total patient days														
Revenue															
	Gross Revenue														
3541.01	1-bed nursing service														
3541.02	2-bed nursing service														
3541.03	4-bed nursing service														
	Total gross revenue														
	Deductions from Gross Revenue														
4541.01	Medicare allowances														
4541.02	Medicaid allowances														
4541.03	Blue Cross allowances														
4541.04	Other contract allowances														
4541.05	Free work and charity														
4541.10	Bad debts														
	Total deductions														
	Net Revenue														
	Variable Operating Expenses														
	Variable Salaries and Wages														
5541.03	Registered nurses														
5541.04	Licensed practical nurses														
5541.05	Nurse aides and orderlies														
5541.09	Ward clerks and others														
5541.10	Employee benefits														
	Total Variable Salaries														

Variable Non-Salary-and-Wage Expenses

6541.15 Office supplies
6541.19 Medical and Surgical supplies
6541.22 Pharmaceuticals
6541.35 Registry fees
6541.50 Other operating expenses
Total variable nonsalary and nonwage Expenses

Total Variable Operating Expenses

Fixed Operating Expenses
Fixed Salaries and Wages
5541.01 Management and supervision
5541.03 Registered nurses
5541.04 Licensed practical nurses
5541.05 Nurse aides and orderlies
5541.09 Ward clerks and others
5541.10 Employee benefits
Total fixed salaries and wages

Fixed Non-Salary-and-Wage Expenses
6541.21 Dues and Subscriptions
6541.25 Depreciation
6541.26 Insurance
6541.27 Equipment leases
6541.28 Training programs
6541.29 Educational travel
6541.30 Recruitment fees, etc.
Total Fixed nonsalary and nonwage expenses

Total Fixed Operating Expenses

Total Fixed and Variable Expenses

Net Operating Contribution

produced and they serve as the multiplicant to the standard rate in order to compute the related monthly revenues and/or expenses.

11. *Standard Variable Revenue Rates*. These rates represent the gross price of the related financial production unit value of each variable revenue item.

12. *Standard Variable Deductions from Revenue Rates*. These standard rates may be expressed in either percentage of total related revenue or in a dollar value per production unit.

13. *Standard Variable Expense Rates*. These rates are usually expressed in the dollar value of each related variable cost item.

14. *Cross-footed Monthly Totals*. Cross-footing of all monthly financial and statistical totals to the annual "total" column helps to assure accuracy and facilitates reader comprehension.

After these key information factors are incorporated in the budget worksheet or spreadsheet, monthly revenue and expense totals are computed by multiplying the standard variable rates by the related monthly volume. To do this manually usually requires less preparation time than programming a microcomputer model. However, after the basic spreadsheet is designed and programmed, the multiplying and adding processes are time consuming, and if the initial end result (i.e., net operating profit) does not meet the desired expectations, changes must be made, and this additional processing of the data will take more time.

The microcomputer spreadsheet methodology, with its simulation capabilities, is the most desirable way of generating a departmental budget, because

1. the computation formulae, which are incorporated in the basic format, assure continuity and accuracy of computation
2. the results can be easily and uniformly reproduced

Most important, the microcomputer spreadsheet approach gives users an opportunity to play "what if" or simulation games. It allows a user to select one or more variables and to conduct sensitivity tests to evaluate the result of changing these variables. For example, what if the volume experiences a 3 percent decrease? or what if the wages were increased 5 percent? or what if the selling price was decreased by 10 dollars? In the highly competitive health care market, selling prices and related costs will be key factors in determining a health care organization's viability and competitiveness. Having the ability to conduct "what if" and sensitivity testings can be essential.

NOTES

1. Robert Kreitner, *Management: A Problem Solving Approach* (Boston: Houghton Mifflin, 1980), 54.

2. American Hospital Association, *The Practice of Planning* (Chicago: American Hospital Association, 1973), 3.

3. Jon B. Jaeger, "The Concept of Corporate Planning," *Health Care Management Review* (Summer 1982): 21–22.

4. Jonathon S. Rakich, Beaufort B. Longest, Jr., and Kurt Darr, *Managing Health Services Organizations* (Philadelphia: Saunders, 1985), 214.

5. Ibid.

6. Peter F. Drucker, *Management: Tasks, Responsibilities, Practices* (New York: Harper & Row, 1974), 94.

7. Herman C. Heiser, *Budgeting: Principles and Practice* (New York: Ronald Press, 1959), 66.

8. Allen G. Herkimer, Jr., *Understanding Hospital Financial Management*, 2d ed. (Rockville, Md.: Aspen, 1986), 48–60.

9. Ibid.

10. Allen G. Herkimer, Jr., *Concepts in Hospital Financial Management* (San Marcos, Tex.: Alfa Management Services, 1970), 87–88.

11. Ibid.

12. Robin E. MacStravic, *Marketing Health Care* (Rockville, Md.: Aspen, 1977), 111.

Chapter 3

Productivity and Production Units

Productivity has been defined as the relationship between the quantity of goods and services produced (the outputs) and the quantity of labor, capital, land, energy, and other resources (the inputs) that produce it.[1]

Productivity is the first test of management's competence; it represents the balance between all factors of production which will give the greatest output for the smallest effort.[2] For its application in the budgetary planning and control process, productivity is defined as the ratio of outputs (production units) to the amount of inputs (resources) required to generate the production units over a specific period of time. Since a department's efficiency is frequently based on its productivity, the selection of the production unit is critical for appropriate planning and control.

CRITERIA FOR SELECTING A DEPARTMENT'S PRODUCTION UNIT

The production unit is the quantitative unit (usually a nondollar value) used to measure the productivity of a health care department, e.g., a laboratory test, radiology exam, surgical case, pound of laundry processed, patient bill processed, etc. If the production unit is knowledgeably selected, the department manager can use it as the basis for calculating the following:

1. productivity (volume) of the department
2. productivity per employee (or per hour)
3. cost per production unit
4. price or charge per production unit

Production units are usually classified into the following two major categories: (1) macro production units and (2) micro production units.[3] When selecting the production unit for a department, it is important that management not limit itself to concentrating on or selecting only one production unit. In many departments, it may be beneficial to use both a macro and a micro unit. For example, an emergency service department manager might find it appropriate to use the following:

- macro production unit: number of E.R. admissions or visits to measure the production of the E.R. admitting staff
- micro production unit: number of E.R. minutes of service to measure the production of the medical and/or nursing staff

The primary criterion for the selection of a department's production unit should be that the selected unit is relevant to the product or service generated by the department or its various sections. Other criteria to be considered are that the production unit is

1. easy to relate to and understand
2. easy to identify, record, and collect
3. easy to trace and audit
4. relatively inexpensive to compute and process

MACRO PRODUCTION UNIT

Macro production units are the most commonly used, because they generally require few or no special studies in order to determine a weighted value. In addition, macro units are relatively easy to identify, collect, and audit.[4]

Macro production units often represent a collection or grouping of related inputs which, when combined, can be identified as a product or a service, such as a patient day, outpatient visit, surgical case, etc. The macro statistic, however, makes no attempt to equate or to measure the amount of resources required to generate the statistic. For example, it would be inequitable to calculate the average cost of an inpatient day and then price the service based on that average cost, because some of the patient days may be accumulated from the intensive care unit (ICU) while others may have been generated in the medical and surgical unit (M&S), the orthopedic unit, or the self-care unit. Each department generating patient days uses different resources, in varying amounts, to care for its patients. However, macro production units can be used for pricing if they are relevant to each other, e.g., ICU to ICU patient days, M&S to M&S patient days, etc.

Macro production units are better than no production unit at all, because they identify what a department produces. However, every department manager is encouraged to identify a unit which attempts to measure the amount of resources required to generate the department's services and to assign a relative weighted value. The macro production unit should be used only when there are no alternatives—and then used with caution.

MICRO PRODUCTION UNIT

The micro production unit, or the relative value unit (RVU), attempts to weigh the relevant relationship between one macro production unit and another, both usually in the same department, e.g., two laboratory tests, etc. This can be accomplished by establishing a basis from which to measure the amount of resources required to produce the units.

For example, assume that a series of time and motion studies have determined that the number of minutes of technical, aide, and clerical (TAC) time required to generate the following macro units is as shown:

Macro Unit	TAC Time
Unit A	10
Unit B	50
Unit C	75

Further assume that the following data represent the volume of macro production units produced by two of the same kinds of departments in two separate hospitals:

Macro Units	Hospital A (number produced)	Hospital B (number produced)
Unit A	130	50
Unit B	50	55
Unit C	10	35
Total units	190	140

At first glance it would appear that Hospital A's department has a greater volume of productivity than Hospital B's, because its total macro production units exceed by 50 the total units produced at Hospital B. The fallacy in concluding this is that no weighted values have been assigned to these production units. By assigning the TAC times as the relative value to the appropriate macro units, they assume a common relativity and are then classified as micro units (or RVUs).

Let us further assume that each department has five full-time equivalent (FTE) employees. A comparative analysis of Hospital A's and Hospital B's departmental productivity follows:

		Hospital A		Hospital B	
Micro Unit	Value	Macro	Micro	Macro	Micro
Unit A	10	130	1,300	50	500
Unit B	50	50	2,500	55	2,750
Unit C	75	10	750	35	2,625
Total units		190	4,550	140	5,875
Macro units per FTE		38	NA	28	NA
Micro units per FTE		NA	910	NA	1,175
Average micro units per macro unit		23.95		41.96	

Using the macro unit to measure productivity, Hospital A's employees appear to be more productive than Hospital B's by 10 units, whereas using the micro production unit methodology, Hospital B's employees have 265 micro units of greater production efficiency. Another conclusion which could be derived from this analysis is that Hospital B is producing, on the average, a more complicated type of service, because its average number of micro units per macro unit is 41.96, which exceeds Hospital A's average of 23.95 by 18.01.

In summary, the use of a micro production unit establishes measurements of relativity between macro units according to the amount of resources required to produce the units. Since much of the distortion in production ratios is eliminated, the micro production unit serves as a reasonably reliable measurement with which to compute a department's total operating expenses and the cost of a department's production unit; it can also serve as the basis for determining the selling price of a department's services.

A comparative list of macro and micro production units used in many health care facilities is displayed in Table 3-1.

Several attempts have been made to create one production unit—a hospital resource unit (HRU)—which could serve as a common unit of measurement for all health services (e.g., laboratory, nursing, housekeeping, etc.). At this writing, these approaches are still in the experimental stages.[5]

One word of caution in selecting a department's production unit: The department manager must select the unit which most appropriately serves the purpose for which it is to be used. For example, a group of departmental production units are mandated by external governing agencies, e.g., Medicare, Medicaid, state rate control commissions, etc. These units are designed to serve whatever purposes the external agencies have selected them for (e.g., payment systems, cost comparisons, etc.), and some mandated production units may not meet the needs of the individual health care institution. While provisions must be made to record and to accumulate these externally prescribed units, the health care facility's management team might determine that other measurements would be more appropriate for their needs and for their internal management information system. Most important is for the facility to use as many production units for a department as is

Table 3-1 Comparative List of Macro and Micro Production Units Commonly Used in Health Care Institutions

Department	Macro Unit	Micro Unit
General Services		
Admitting offices	number of admissions	types of admissions
Billing and collections	number of billings	types of billings
Dietary	meals served	weighted meals served
Cafeteria	number of FTEs*	weighted meals served
Computer services	number of reports	computer time
Plant operations	square footage	hours of service
Human resources	salaries and wages	number of employees
Housekeeping	square footage	hours of service
Medical records	number of discharges	types of discharges
Social services	number of visits	weighted visits
Patient Care Services		
Nursing	patient day	hours of service or type of nursing care
Laboratory	tests	relative values (RVU)
Radiology	examinations	relative values (RVU)
Operating room	surgical cases	OR person minutes† or OR minutes
Delivery room	deliveries	delivery room minutes
Anesthesiology	cases	anesthesia minutes
Physical therapy	treatments	relative values (RVU)
Respiratory therapy	treatments	relative values (RVU)
Recovery or postoperative room	cases	person-minutes
Emergency services	visits or cases	person-minutes

*The number of FTE (full-time equivalent) employees is computed by dividing the number of paid hours by the number of hours during the period. For example, the average employee is paid for 52 40-hour weeks. Based on a year's data, the value of one FTE is calculated as follows: 52 weeks × 40 hours = 2,080 hours.
†Operating room (OR) person-minutes, as compared to OR minutes, are computed by multiplying the number of OR minutes by the number of paid personnel, e.g., 30 OR minutes × 3 paid personnel = 90 OR person-minutes.

necessary to effectively and efficiently evaluate, manage, and control the department. It is advisable to limit the number of production units for the budgetary planning and control process to four or less whenever possible.

HISTORICAL DATA AND THEIR USES

After a department's production unit has been identified, the department's historical data constitute the most accurate and reliable source for beginning the volume forecasting process, which is discussed in detail in Chapter 4.

In addition to volume forecasting, among the most meaningful uses of a production unit are the profitability/productivity (P/P) trend analyses. The P/P trend analyses evaluate the profitability and the productivity of a department, a departmental section, and/or a full-time equivalent (FTE) employee and production unit. P/P studies can be conducted using the following types of data: (1) historical, (2) concurrent, and (3) future.

Historical trends are established by collecting financial and statistical data (see Exhibit 3-1) and plotting them on graphs (see Figures 3-1, 3-2, and 3-3). P/P studies based on historical data display to the analyst what the profitability and productivity trends have been. These same trend analyses can be continued on a concurrent basis and/or used as the basis on which to project future goals.

An analysis of the P/P trend illustrated in Figure 3-1 reveals that while total departmental revenue parallels and exceeds the departmental expenses, the total production unit trend line does not maintain a similar pattern, the first indication that something may be wrong. The revenue per production unit (RVU) in Figure 3-2 is greater than the unit expense for only two out of the five years. This adverse pattern is highlighted in Figure 3-3, which identifies a steady decline in units per FTE, from 109,588 per year in 19x1 to 44,084 in 19x5.

In each of the figures, historical data were collected and plotted on graphs to facilitate the analyst's recognition of the trends. The analyst, usually the department manager, must fully understand the source and the meaning of the data collected. The use of graphs reduces the columns of numbers to a relatively simple form for reading, analyzing, and interpreting these data.

STANDARD PRICE DETERMINATION

Knowing the cost of any service a department produces is vitally important, and since the production unit selected best represents, in quantitative terms, a department's production, this same unit should be used in determining both the cost and the selling price of the service.

Production unit cost can be calculated based on either historical or budgeted costs. However, for the purposes of establishing the selling price of a production unit, it is advisable to use the department's total budgeted expenses, both direct expenses and those allocated to the department. This type of cost analysis is usually done after the entire budget has been subjected to the cost-finding process so as to determine the allocated expenses of non-revenue-producing departments as well as the service department's direct costs. The total costs are then divided by the total budgeted production units to determine the cost per unit.

Using Hometown Memorial Hospital's clinical laboratory data for year 19x5 (see Exhibit 3-1), the average cost per relative unit (RVU) is calculated as

Exhibit 3-1 Sample Comparative Statistical Data

Hometown Memorial Hospital
Hometown, U.S.A.

Clinical Laboratory Department
Comparative Statistical Data
for the Years 19x1 Through 19x5

Description	19x1	19x2	19x3	19x4	19x5
Laboratory tests	712,320	736,848	529,062	480,880	511,373
Relative value units (RVUs)	1,780,800	1,842,120	2,010,438	2,163,964	2,352,315
Patient days	10,176	10,234	10,986	11,572	10,941
RVUs per patient day	175	180	183	187	215
Lab tests per patient day	70	72	48	42	47
RVUs per lab test	2.5	2.5	3.8	4.5	4.6
Gross revenue	$4,452,000.00	$4,789,512.00	$5,528,705.00	$5,950,901.00	$6,586,482.00
Net revenue	$4,006,800.00	$4,236,876.00	$4,825,051.00	$5,085,315.00	$5,763,171.00
Net expense	$3,917,760.00	$4,328,982.00	$4,724,529.00	$5,193,513.00	$5,880,788.00
Net profit (loss)	$89,040.00	($92,106.00)	$100,522.00	($108,198.00)	($117,617.00)
Number of FTEs	6.5	8.1	8.2	9.2	11.6
Number of paid hours	13,520	16,848	17,056	19,136	24,128
Number RVUs per FTE	273,969	227,422	245,175	235,213	202,786
Number of RVUs per paid hour	132	109	118	113	97
Number lab tests per FTE	109,588	90,969	64,520	52,270	44,084
Number lab tests per paid hour	53	44	31	25	21
Gross revenue per FTE	$684,923.08	$591,297.78	$674,232.32	$646,837.07	$567,800.17
Gross revenue per paid hour	$329.29	$284.28	$324.15	$310.98	$272.98
Gross revenue per RVU	$2.50	$2.60	$2.75	$2.75	$2.80

Exhibit 3-1 continued

Description	19x1	19x2	19x3	19x4	19x5
Gross revenue per patient day	$437.50	$468.00	$503.25	$514.25	$602.00
Gross revenue per lab test	$6.25	$6.50	$10.45	$12.38	$12.88
Net revenue per FTE	$616,430.77	$523,071.11	$588,420.85	$552,751.63	$496,825.09
Net revenue per paid hour	$296.36	$251.48	$282.89	$265.75	$238.86
Net revenue per RVU	$2.25	$2.30	$2.40	$2.35	$2.45
Net revenue per patient day	$393.75	$414.00	$439.20	$439.45	$526.75
Net revenue per lab test	$5.63	$5.75	$9.12	$10.58	$11.27
Net expense per FTE	$602,732.31	$534,442.22	$576,162.07	$564,512.28	$506,964.48
Net expense per paid hour	$289.78	$256.94	$277.00	$271.40	$243.73
Net expense per RVU	$2.20	$2.35	$2.35	$2.40	$2.50
Net expense per patient day	$385.00	$423.00	$430.05	$448.80	$537.50
Net expense per lab test	$5.50	$5.88	$8.93	$10.80	$11.50
Net profit (loss) per FTE	$13,698.46	($11,371.11)	$12,258.78	($11,760.65)	($10,139.40)
Net profit (loss) per paid hour	$6.59	($5.47)	$5.89	($5.65)	($4.87)
Net profit (loss) per RVU	$0.05	($0.05)	$0.05	($0.05)	($0.05)
Net profit (loss) per patient day	$8.75	($9.00)	$9.15	($9.35)	($10.75)
Net profit (loss) per lab test	$0.13	($0.13)	$0.19	($0.23)	($0.23)

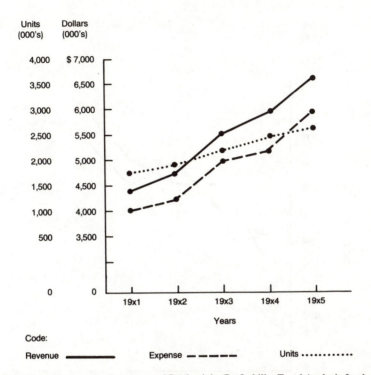

Figure 3-1 Clinical Laboratory Departmental Productivity/Profitability Trend Analysis for the Years 19x1 through 19x5

follows. The net operating expenses equal $5,880,788 and the total production units (RVUs) equal 2,352,315.

$$\frac{\text{Total departmental expenses}}{\text{Total production units}} = \text{average cost per production unit}$$

or

$$\frac{\$\ 5,880,788}{2,352,315} = \$2.50$$

This average cost will serve as the basis from which to establish the selling price of each RVU produced by the clinical laboratory. For example, assume that the hospital wants to generate a 25 percent markup on costs. The selling price per RVU would be computed as follows:

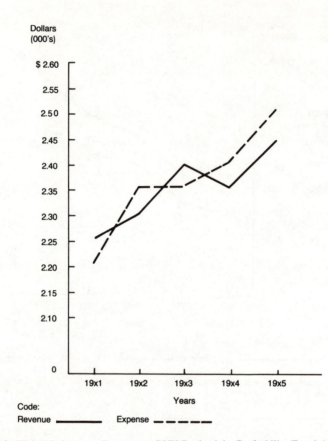

Dollars
(000's)

Code:
Revenue ————   Expense — — — —

Figure 3-2 Clinical Laboratory Department RVU Productivity/Profitability Trend Analysis for the Years 19x1 through 19x5

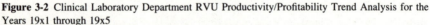

Average cost per production unit (RVU) + desired percent of markup on cost-selling price per RVU

or

$2.50   +   (.25 × $2.50)   =   selling price per RVU

or

$2.50   + $ .625   = $3.125

The computed RVU selling price ($3.125) can then be used as the factor to be multiplied by the RVU value of each clinical laboratory test so as to determine the ultimate selling price for each test, as follows:

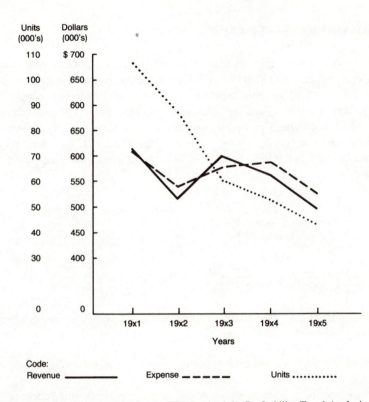

Figure 3-3 Clinical Laboratory Department FTE Productivity/Profitability Trend Analysis for the Years 19x1 through 19x5

Test Description	Value	Unit Price	Test Price
Total cholesterol	10.0	$3.125	$31.25
Platelet count	14.0	3.125	43.75
Blood culture	9.0	3.125	28.13

This costing and pricing system is unique, because it is extremely flexible, especially when the RVU values of each laboratory test are stored in the computer system. Since these values remain relatively constant over a reasonable length of time, the selling price of the RVU needs minimal adjustment after the budget and the initial pricing structure have been determined.

To be competitive, it may be necessary to selectively price certain laboratory tests. For example, if the laboratory wants to establish an especially competitive price on any test, such as a complete blood count (CBC), Pap smear, or SMA-12, the price can be locked into the computer as a ''special'' price, while all other tests are priced at the established average price per RVU.

STANDARD VARIABLE COSTS

The variable budget process requires not only standard prices for its production units, it also demands a standard cost for each variable expense item or group of items. The standard variable expense rate is computed by using *only* the department's direct variable historical or budgeted expense totals. For example, assuming that Hometown Memorial Hospital's clinical laboratory expenses for chemicals and reagents during the year 19x5 were $682,171, the standard variable (historical) cost per RVU for chemicals and reagents would be computed as follows:

$$\frac{\text{Total annual expense}}{\text{Total annual volume (RVUs)}} = \text{standard variable cost per RVU}$$

or

$$\frac{\$682,171}{2,352,315} = \$ .29$$

To compute a budgeted standard variable cost of chemicals and reagents, the following approach could be used:

Historical standard cost + anticipated inflationary increase = budget standard variable cost

Assuming the inflation rato is anticipated to be 10 percent, this becomes

$$\$ .29 + (.10 \times .29) = \text{budget standard variable cost}$$

or

$$\$ .29 + \$ .03 = \$ .32$$

Standard costs are usually computed for *each* variable expense item. This approach allows the department manager to analyze each expense item for any deviation of the actual performance from the budgeted standard. In some instances, a group of like expense items, such as food, may be grouped together, but a certain degree of control is lost for the sake of convenience.

PRODUCTION STANDARDS

Production standards are the desired quantitative results (outputs) generated through the use of a specific amount of resources (inputs). Production standards are usually expressed in relation to the amount of employee time required to generate the output, such as the number of production units per paid hour, work hour, or FTE.

Assume the department manager of Hometown Memorial Hospital's clinical laboratory wants to generate 100 RVUs per paid technician hour on a projected annual production unit volume of 2,556,966. In this case, the staffing requirements could be computed as follows:

Step 1:

$$\frac{\text{Volume of units}}{\text{Number of calendar days}} = \text{average units per calendar day}$$

or

$$\frac{2,556,966}{365} = 7,005 \text{ units}$$

Step 2:

$$\frac{\text{Average units per calendar day}}{\text{Hourly production standard}} = \text{employee hours required per calendar day}$$

or

$$\frac{7,005}{100} = 70 \text{ hours}$$

Step 3:

$$\frac{\text{Employee hours required per calendar day}}{\text{Average employee hours per calendar day}} = \text{number of required FTEs}$$

or

$$\frac{70}{8} = 8.75 \text{ FTEs}$$

Production standards are usually established by management through the use of management engineering studies but the department manager may take an equally effective approach by using historical production levels and adding the desired increase in productivity. For example:

Historical RVUs per paid hour + desired increase = new production standard per paid hour

or

97 RVUs per paid hour + 10 increase = new production standard per paid hour

or

$$97 + 10 = 107$$

If this approach is used, it *must* be calculated in cooperation with the personnel who will be evaluated by these production standards. These production standards are often successful and useful because the employees, as well as the department manager, understand how they were computed and therefore tend to more readily accept and use them.

To illustrate how this production standard may be used, assume that the Hometown Memorial Hospital's clinical laboratory manager established a production standard of 107 RVUs per paid hour, or 856 RVUs per person (eight-hour) day. Using the 19x5 total RVUs listed in Exhibit 3-1, it can be assumed that the department would have required 7.5 paid technicians per calendar day, computed as follows:

Step 1:

$$\frac{\text{Total RVUs}}{\text{Total calendar days}} = \text{RVUs per calendar day}$$

or

$$\frac{2,352,315}{365} = 6,445$$

Step 2:

$$\frac{\text{RVUs per calendar day}}{\substack{\text{Production standard per} \\ \text{paid 8-hour day}}} = \text{average number required FTEs}$$

or

$$\frac{6,445}{107 \times 8} = 7.5 \text{ FTEs}$$

The methodology used to establish production standards is not as important as the understanding and acceptance of these standards by both management and employees. No matter how exact a standard is, it becomes meaningful only if it is used knowledgeably by the persons for whom it is intended. A standard arrived at scientifically but rejected by management and employees is useless; one in whose development and establishment everyone was involved not only will be accepted but also used. If the standard proves inadequate, refinement and accuracy can always be improved—after acceptance is assured.[6]

NOTES

1. Allen G. Herkimer, Jr., *Understanding Hospital Financial Management*, 2d ed. (Rockville, Md.: Aspen, 1986), 91.

2. Peter Drucker, *Management Tasks, Responsibilities, Practices* (New York: Harper & Row, 1973), 77–78.

3. Herkimer, *Understanding Hospital Financial Management*, 90–94.

4. Ibid.

5. Allen G. Herkimer, Jr., "Treatment Degree: A Standard Unit of Measure for All Components of the Health Care Industry," *Healthcare Financial Management*, March 1972; Allen G. Herkimer, Jr., "The HRU—Measuring Input to Find Productivity," *Healthcare Financial Management*, February 1976; Allen G. Herkimer, Jr., et al., "HRU: A Standard Measurement for Hospital Productivity," *Topics in Health Care Financing: Improving Productivity* (Winter 1977).

6. Allen G. Herkimer, Jr., *Developing Production Standards for Physician-Directed Hospital Departments* (Bridgeport, Conn.: University of Bridgeport, 1972), 38–39.

Volume Forecasting

4

After the department's mission, goals, objectives, and expense classification have been decided on and a representative production unit (or units) has been selected, the next step is to develop a volume forecast for the budget year. (The term *activity level* is sometimes used in lieu of *volume forecast*.)[1] The volume forecast attempts to predict, in quantitative terms, what a department and/or a health care institution expects to produce over a specific period of time.

Volume forecasting is so critical to the credibility of any budget that it has been termed the keystone step in the budgetary planning and control process.[2] A health care institution's budget is only as good as its volume forecast.

FORECASTING METHODOLOGIES

The production unit volume forecast is the most reasonable "guesstimate" which a knowledgeable forecaster is able to develop using whatever tools and resources are available. Several highly sophisticated formulae exist (e.g., multiple regression analysis, exponential smoothing, and other quantitative computer programs) for developing the volume forecast, but even these cannot forecast all the variables caused by human and natural elements in the operating environment.

There is no magic formula that will accurately forecast the exact volume of work a department will produce during any given period of time. Perhaps the most reliable resource in volume forecasting is the intuition and common sense of knowledgeable individuals.[3] For the purpose of discussion, the "least squares" forecasting methodology is presented in this chapter. The reader, however, is encouraged to research and test a variety of computer forecasting models, because they make excellent management tools and assist the forecasting process.

In addition to selecting the forecasting methodology to be used, the following key resources should be considered during the forecasting process:

- external and internal competition
- governmental and third party policies
- departmental goals and objectives
- new services and capital expenditures
- historical data and trends
- other known facts and rumors

While these key resources will have varying degrees of impact on the volume forecast, all should be considered, evaluated, and provided for in the forecast. For example, a rumor may be circulated within the service area about another health care facility which is contemplating the installation of a new type of service. It is important that the rumor be investigated, because if the new service is in fact installed, it could have adverse effects on the budgeting institution's planning process and operations.

Third party purchasers of health care, especially the federal and state governments (e.g., Medicare, Medicaid, etc.), are constantly issuing new regulations which affect the ways that health care providers are paid for services or the ways those costs not covered by their programs are identified. Staying aware of these ever-changing regulations and policies is a full-time job, but most health care facilities cannot afford to pay an individual for this purpose alone. The CEO, CFO, and budget director must confer with the institution's auditing firm so as to incorporate into the system provisions for complying with all of the latest regulations.

Two major payment system developments which will have a lasting effect on the health care industry for some time to come involve the use of diagnosis related groups (DRGs) and managed health care contracts (sometimes referred to as "risk-based" contracts).

Medicare's DRG prospective payment system is based on the diagnosis for which a patient is admitted to the health care facility. Since the institution is paid a fixed amount per diagnosis, it is imperative that the institution record and project its revenues based on the number and distribution of the type(s) of DRGs.

Managed health care contracts, such as those negotiated by health maintenance organizations (HMOs), usually pay the health care providers based on a capitation rate. This rate is usually a monthly payment made to the provider regardless of whether or not the patient (member) receives any health care service during the month. Again, it is imperative that the health care institution record and project its related revenues based on the distribution of contracted services at their respective rates and the related volume of subscribers.

In many health care facilities, the traditional fee-for-service type of payment system still prevails. Many health care institutions may have as many as four different types of payment systems, such as fee-for-service, per diem, per case, and per capita.

A fee-for-service payment system identifies and charges only for the specific type(s) of service the patient receives, while per diem (day) and per case systems pay the provider a fixed amount for the day or the case, regardless of the amount of services rendered to the patient. A per capita system, commonly used by HMOs, pays the provider a fixed amount, usually on a monthly basis, whether the member receives any health care services or not. The latter three payment methods are risk-based contracts, while the only risk in the fee-for-service system is whether the provider has priced the service accurately so as not to charge less than the cost of the service.

This variety of payment systems, coupled with the many different rates for each, requires the health care institution to collect a comprehensive statistical record by the volume of services and by the various types of purchaser payment systems and their contract rates.

For the purpose of simplification, we shall develop a case study of the medical and surgical nursing department of Hometown Memorial Hospital. The case study will consider only three types of nursing services; it will examine the way that each is paid based on the types of room accommodations.

Other considerations to include in the volume forecasting process are the department's goals and objectives, together with any anticipated capital expenditures and new services. Chapter 5 reviews the capital expenditure planning process.

HISTORICAL DATA AND TRENDS

If there has been no significant change in either the internal or external environment, the department's historical data and trends provide the most accurate and reliable source for starting the volume forecasting.[4] Trends can be identified with three years of data, but five years of data may identify a more meaningful trend, as illustrated in the time-series chart in Table 4-1. These data may be further refined and analyzed by displaying them graphically, as illustrated in Figure 4-1.

Table 4-1 Medical and Surgical Patient Days for the Years 19x1 through 19x5

Year	Patient Days
19x1	57,488
19x2	55,571
19x3	53,016
19x4	52,377
19x5	54,326*

*Estimate: 8 months actual and 4 months estimated.

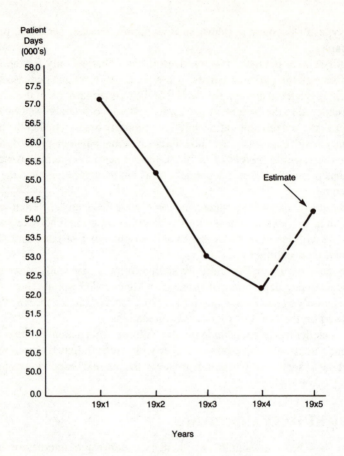

Figure 4-1 Graphic Analysis of Medical and Surgical Patient Days for the Years 19x1 through 19x5

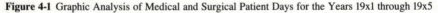

As in most budgeting programs, the current year's actual data are incomplete; consequently, an annualization process was applied. In the above time-series table, the current year 19x5 has been annualized using eight months actual and four months estimated patient days to arrive at 54,326 total patient days. The annualization process is reviewed later in this chapter.

MONTHLY VOLUME DISTRIBUTION

Several methodologies can be used to compensate for seasonal volume variations in the monthly distribution of the institution's product(s). The most commonly used method is called the *even month distribution process*. For example, assume that the annual volume forecast was 55,905 patient days. The monthly distribution would be computed as follows:

$$\frac{\text{Total patient days}}{\text{Total calendar months}} = \text{monthly patient days per calendar month}$$

$$\frac{55,905}{12} = 4,659 \text{ patient days per calendar month}$$

Using this approach, each month's volume would be calculated at 4,659, regardless of the number of calendar days in the month.

Another monthly distribution method is based upon the number of calendar days in each month, computed as follows:

$$\frac{\text{Total patient days}}{\text{Total calendar days}} = \text{daily patient days}$$

$$\frac{55,905}{365} = 153 \text{ patient days per calendar day}$$

Using the *calendar day method*, the patient day volume is distributed by multiplying the average patient day total (153) by the number of calendar days in the month. This approach usually is more acceptable than the even month distribution model, but the most universally accepted method is the *percentage distribution method* (see Table 4-2).

The percentage distribution method for monthly volume forecasting uses the previous and/or the present year's actual monthly distribution and calculates the monthly percentage of the total annual volume. For example, if January's actual volume was 4,800 patient days and the annual patient day total was 54,326, January's monthly percentage distribution would be 0.088356 (see Table 4-2). For the purpose of this case study, we suggest that the percentage distribution method be used. However, another variation of the percentage distribution method is illustrated in Table 4-3. This approach uses two years: the previous year and the present year.

The two years' monthly volumes are all added together and the total is used as the base for calculating the monthly percentages, as illustrated in the following example (see Table 4-3). Suppose the previous year's total number of patient days in January was 4,624 and the present year's total was 4,800, resulting in a monthly total of 9,424. This number is then divided by the two-year patient day total of 106,703, resulting in a January monthly percentage distribution of .0883199.

To further assist the forecaster, Table 4-4 is a capacity and occupancy analysis of the medical and surgical patient days of Hometown Memorial Hospital.

Table 4-2 One-Year Monthly Percentage Distribution of Medical and Surgical Patient Days for the Year Ending December 31, 19x5

Month	Patient Days	Percent Distribution
January	4,800	.088356
February	4,291	.078986
March	4,530	.083385
April	4,609	.084840
May	4,546	.083680
June	4,291	.078986
July	4,132	.076059
August	4,390	.080808
September	4,609	.084840
October	4,927	.090693
November	4,751	.087450
December	4,750	.081913
Total	54,326	1.000000

Table 4-3 Two-Year Monthly Percentage Distribution of Medical and Surgical Patient Days for the Fiscal Years Ending December 31, 19x4 and 19x5

Month	Previous Year 19x4	Present Year 19x5	Two-Year Total	Percent Distribution
January	4,624	4,800	9,424	.0883199
February	4,085	4,291	8,376	.0784982
March	4,363	4,430	8,893	.0833434
April	4,399	4,609	9,008	.0844212
May	4,347	4,546	8,893	.0833434
June	4,085	4,291	8,376	.0784982
July	3,980	4,132	8,112	.0760241
August	4,190	4,390	8,580	.0804101
September	4,401	4,609	9,010	.0844399
October	4,745	4,927	9,672	.0906447
November	4,577	4,751	9,328	.0874202
December	4,581	4,450	9,031	.0846367
Total	52,377	54,326	106,703	100.0000000

LEAST SQUARES FORECASTING METHODOLOGY

One of the most commonly used mathematical formulae to identify trend lines and to develop volume forecasts is the *least squares* or *simple regression method*. This method assumes that if a straight line is "fitted" to either graphic or time

Table 4-4 Capacity and Occupancy Analysis of Medical and Surgical Patient Days for the Year Ending December 31, 19x5

Month	Calendar Days	Capacity (175 beds)	Patient Days	Percent Occupancy
January	31	5,425	4,800	88%
February	28	4,900	4,291	88
March	31	5,425	4,530	84
April	30	5,250	4,609	88
May	31	5,425	4,546	84
June	30	5,250	4,291	82
July	31	5,425	4,132	76
August	31	5,425	4,390	81
September	30	5,250	4,609*	88
October	31	5,425	4,927*	91
November	30	5,250	4,751*	90
December	31	5,425	4,450*	82
Total	365	63,875	54,326*	85

*Estimated and annualized

series data, it will serve as a reasonable trend line to project the subsequent year's volume. The least squares method uses a relatively simple mathematical formula, but while it is a reasonably accurate way of fitting a trend line to historical data, the results must be evaluated and tempered with a healthy dose of "common sense and knowledgeable judgment."[5]

The method of least squares is a mathematical device which places a line through a series of plotted points in such a way that the sum of the squares of the deviations of the actual points above and below the trend line is at a minimum. This is as near as is convenient to getting a line of the least deviations, and is therefore accepted as the "line of best fits."[6] The least square formula is illustrated in Table 4-5.

Note that the least squares method requires an odd number of years of historical data in order to identify a midpoint year. In this illustration, the midpoint year (19x3) is represented by the five-year average of 54,555 patient days. To determine the "line of best fits," the annual trend increment (450) is subtracted for 19x1 and 19x2 and added for 19x4 and 19x5. To arrive at the forecast of 55,905 for the budget year 19x6, three annual increments were added to the five-year average, as follows:

Average year (19x3) = 54,555
Future year (19x6):
    54,555 + (450 × 3) = future patient days

or

    54,555 + 1,350 = 55,905

Table 4-5 Least Squares Worksheet Applied to Five-Year Medical and Surgical Patient Days to Project Patient Days for the Budget Year Ending December 31, 19x6

Year (X = no. of years)	Actual Patient Days (Y = no. of patient days)	Time Deviation of Each Year from Middle Year (x)	Square of x Deviation (x²)	xY
19x1	57,488	−2	4	− 114,976
19x2	55,571	−1	1	− 55,571
19x3	53,016	0	0	0
19x4	52,377	+1	1	+ 52,377
19x5	54,326	+2	4	+108,652
Total	272,778	0	10	+ 45,037

Average = Y/X = 272,778/5 = 54,555

Annual Increment = xY/x² = +45,037/10 = 450

The actual patient days and their trend ordinates (see Table 4-6) are plotted on the graph in Figure 4-2.

The monthly distribution (see Table 4-5) of the budgeted patient day volume (55,905) is computed based on the present year's monthly distribution (computed in Table 4-2).

Like most health care departments, Hometown Memorial Hospital's medical and surgical routine nursing services department has more than one type of service. It has 1-bed, 2-bed, and 4-bed nursing services. Consequently, in addition to the budgeted monthly total patient day forecast (see Table 4-7), a monthly patient day forecast must be made for *each* of these types of service. These forecasts, based on historical data and other known facts, are illustrated in Tables 4-8 and 4-9.

Table 4-6 Application of Annual Increment to Project Future Patient Days Based on Computations in Table 4-5

Year	Average or Midpoint	+/−	Annual Increment	=	Trend Ordinates
19x1	54,555	+	(450 × −2)	=	53,655
19x2	54,555	+	(450 × −1)	=	54,105
19x3	54,555	+	0	=	54,555
19x4	54,555	+	(450 × +1)	=	55,005
19x5	54,555	+	(450 × +2)	=	55,455
Future Projections:					
19x6	54,555	+	(450 × +3)	=	55,905
19x7	54,555	+	(450 × +4)	=	56,355
19x8	54,555	+	(450 × +5)	=	56,805

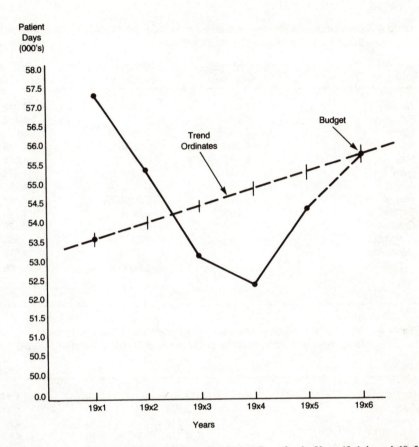

Figure 4-2 Graphic Analysis of Medical and Surgical Patient Days for the Years 19x1 through 19x5 and the Projected Budget Year Ending December 31, 19x6

One word of caution: The monthly percentage distribution method of forecasting is appropriate only if there have been no major changes in the institution's delivery services, e.g., new services, losses or additions of physicians, etc. If any significant changes have occurred, then appropriate adjustments must be made to the monthly distributions in order to compensate for these changes.

PLOTTING THE VOLUME FORECAST

After the volume forecast has been completed (see Table 4-8) to the satisfaction of the department manager and the budget director, the production units should be

Table 4-7 Computation of Monthly Distribution of Medical and Surgical Patient Days for the Budget Year Ending December 31, 19x6

Month	Present Year Patient Days	Percent Distribution	Budget Year Patient Days
January	4,800	0.088356	4,940
February	4,291	0.078986	4,416
March	4,530	0.083385	4,662
April	4,609	0.084840	4,743
May	4,546	0.083680	4,678
June	4,291	0.078986	4,416
July	4,132	0.076059	4,252
August	4,390	0.080808	4,517
September	4,609	0.084840	4,743
October	4,927	0.090693	5,070
November	4,751	0.087454	4,889
December	4,450	0.081913	4,579
Total	54,326	1.000000	55,905

Table 4-8 Monthly Distribution of Medical and Surgical Patient Days by Types of Nursing Service Accommodations for the Year Ending December 31, 19x6

Month	1-Bed	2-Bed	4-Bed	Total
January	705	2,881	1,354	4,940
February	630	2,576	1,210	4,416
March	666	2,716	1,280	4,662
April	675	2,772	1,296	4,743
May	666	2,732	1,280	4,678
June	630	2,576	1,210	4,416
July	604	2,487	1,161	4,252
August	643	2,639	1,235	4,517
September	675	2,772	1,296	4,743
October	721	2,965	1,384	5,070
November	698	2,852	1,339	4,889
December	651	2,678	1,250	4,579
Total	7,964	32,646	15,295	55,905

identified and plotted along the top of the variable budget spreadsheet in each month's column, as displayed in Exhibit 4-1. The use of the volume forecast is discussed throughout the balance of this book.

Table 4-9 Detailed Monthly Distribution Worksheet of Medical and Surgical Patient Days by Accommodation for the Year Ending December 31, 19x6

Description	January	February	March	April	May	June	July	August	September	October	November	December	Total
Number of calendar days	31	28	31	30	31	30	31	31	30	31	30	31	365
Number of Beds													
1-bed rooms	25	25	25	25	25	25	25	25	25	25	25	25	25
2-bed rooms	102	102	102	102	102	102	102	102	102	102	102	102	102
4-bed rooms	48	48	48	48	48	48	48	48	48	48	48	48	48
Total number of beds	175	175	175	175	175	175	175	175	175	175	175	175	175
Capacity by Rooms													
1-bed room capacity	775	700	775	750	775	750	775	775	750	775	750	775	9125
2-bed room capacity	3162	2856	3162	3060	3162	3060	3162	3162	3060	3162	3060	3162	37230
4-bed room capacity	1488	1344	1488	1440	1488	1440	1488	1488	1440	1488	1440	1488	17520
Total capacity by rooms	5425	4900	5425	5250	5425	5250	5425	5425	5250	5425	5250	5425	63875
Monthly occupancy rate	0.91	0.9	0.86	0.9	0.86	0.84	0.78	0.83	0.9	0.93	0.93	0.84	
Budgeted Patient Days													
1-bed room patient days	705	630	666	675	666	630	604	643	675	721	698	651	7964
2-bed room patient days	2881	2576	2716	2772	2732	2576	2487	2639	2772	2965	2852	2678	32646
4-bed room patient days	1354	1210	1280	1296	1280	1210	1161	1235	1296	1384	1339	1250	15295
Total budgeted patient days	4940	4416	4662	4743	4678	4416	4252	4517	4743	5070	4889	4579	55905
Budgeted Occupancy Rate													
1-bed room occupancy rate	91%	90%	86%	90%	86%	84%	78%	83%	90%	93%	93%	84%	87%
2-bed room occupancy rate	91%	90%	86%	91%	86%	84%	79%	83%	91%	94%	93%	85%	88%
4-bed room occupancy rate	91%	90%	86%	90%	86%	84%	78%	83%	90%	93%	93%	84%	87%
Average budgeted occupancy	91%	90%	86%	90%	86%	84%	78%	83%	90%	93%	93%	84%	88%

Exhibit 4-1 Departmental Variable Budget

Hometown Memorial Hospital
Hometown, U.S.A.

Department: Medical and Surgical Routine Nursing

Account Number	Description	Standard Rate	January	February	March	April	May	June	July	August	September	October	November	December	Total
	Volume:														
	1-bed patient days		705	630	666	675	666	630	604	643	675	721	698	651	7,964
	2-bed patient days		2,881	2,576	2,716	2,772	2,732	2,576	2,487	2,639	2,772	2,965	2,852	2,678	32,646
	4-bed patient days		1,354	1,210	1,280	1,296	1,280	1,210	1,161	1,235	1,296	1,384	1,339	1,250	15,295
	Total patient days		4,940	4,416	4,662	4,743	4,678	4,416	4,252	4,517	4,743	5,070	4,889	4,579	55,905

Gross Revenue
3541.01 1-bed nursing service
3541.02 2-bed nursing service
3541.03 4-bed nursing service
   Total gross revenue

Deductions from Gross Revenue
4541.01 Medicare allowances
4541.02 Medicaid allowances
4541.03 Blue Cross allowances
4541.04 Other contract allowances
4531.05 Free work and charity
4541.10 Bad debts
   Total deductions

Net Revenue

NOTES

1. Corine T. Norgaard, *Management Accounting* (Englewood Cliffs, N.J.: Prentice-Hall, 1985), 235–36

2. Allen G. Herkimer, Jr., *Understanding Hospital Financial Management,* 2d ed. (Rockville, Md.: Aspen, 1986), 117.

3. Ibid., 122.

4. Ibid., 122–23.

5. Ibid., 133–35.

6. John R. Rigglemann and Ira N. Frisbee, *Business Statistics* (New York: McGraw-Hill, 1938), 297–98.

Capital Expenditure Planning

5

The investment decisions of whether to buy, no-buy, lease, or no-lease in a capital expenditure may be the most important a department manager has to make. When the decision is made and the contract is signed, the department and the health care facility are committed to a pattern or route of financial demands, managerial styles, production techniques, service selection—even geographical location—for an extended period of time.[1]

Capital expenditure planning has been defined as the allocation of capital to investment proposals whose benefits are to be realized in the future. Because the future benefits are not known with certainty, investment proposals necessarily involve risks. Consequently, they should be evaluated in relation to their expected return and the incremental risk they add to the health care institution as a whole, for these are the factors that affect the facility's financial viability.[2]

Typically, capital expenditures involve a current investment in a capital asset with a useful life of one or more years. This suggests that an investment in any asset with a useful life of less than a year falls into the realm of working capital management, whereas any asset with a useful life of more than one year involves capital planning. Frequently, there is a great deal of overlap. For example, assume that a new pharmacy delivery system calls for both a remodeled stockroom and distribution centers and an increase in the investment of the pharmaceutical inventory. An investment proposal of this nature must be evaluated as a single package, not as an investment in a fixed asset (the remodeled stockroom and distribution centers) and in a current asset (the inventory). Consequently, the total investment must be considered as a single capital expenditure.[3]

For the purpose of this presentation, a capital expenditure is defined as any one or group of items acquired that will have a long-term (usually more than one year) impact on the type(s) of service rendered by the facility and whose total investment exceeds a financial limit established either by the governing board or the manage-

81

ment team. Additionally, provisions, revenues, expenses, depreciation, etc., for the new capital expenditure must be included in the current year's budget, and an appropriate production unit must be identified to measure the investment's productivity and profitability. In order to facilitate in the project's performance evaluation and control process, a separate program or project budget for the new capital investment is frequently developed.

CLASSIFICATIONS OF CAPITAL EXPENDITURES

Capital expenditures are classified in the following categories:

1. land
2. land improvements
3. buildings
4. fixed equipment
5. major movable equipment
6. minor equipment

Land is a capital expenditure which can either appreciate or depreciate in value. No provision for depreciation of land may be accounted for in the facility's statement of operations (profit and loss statement).

Land improvements, represented by improvements made to land, including sidewalks, parking lots, driveways, fencing, and shrubbery, are depreciable as operating expenses.[4]

Buildings are capital expenditures which house the facility's operations and are usually depreciated over a time period ranging from 20 to 30 years. The exact length of depreciable time is dependent upon the type of construction, e.g., wood, masonry, steel, etc.

Fixed equipment, such as plumbing, wiring, etc., is frequently included in the total cost of the building. In order to recover the fixed equipment investment over a shorter time period, the fixed equipment portion of the building costs is identified and separated and another depreciation schedule is developed. The depreciable life of fixed equipment usually ranges from 12 to 20 years, as compared to 20 to 30 years for buildings.

Major movable equipment has the following characteristics:

1. The units are easily identified and moved from one place to another.
2. The cost of each unit is sufficiently large to justify the additional expense to control by means of a subsidiary plant ledger.
3. Each unit's individuality and size are sufficient to make control feasible by means of identification tags and numbers.[5]

Although some facilities may place a minimum length of useful life and/or minimum value on movable equipment (e.g., three years and $500), the equipment might be significant enough (e.g., a desk calculator costing $250) to justify logging the equipment in the plant ledger and taking the total cost off as a one-year depreciation expense. This requires establishing a permanent record of the equipment in the plant ledger and allows the investment to be recovered as depreciation in one year. Regardless of the approach suggested in this text, the depreciation methodology used will be one based upon the policies established by the health care institution's Governing Board.

Minor equipment has the following characteristics:

1. The units have no fixed location within the facility and are subject to requisition and use by various departments.
2. Each unit is relatively small in size and cost.
3. There are a large quantity of units in use and they are subject to storeroom control.
4. Each unit has a maximum useful life of three years.[6]

Usually, the initial cost of minor equipment (e.g., wastebaskets, bedpans, surgical instruments, etc.) is depreciated over a period of three years, and all subsequent purchases are recorded as expenses to the requisitioning departments.[7]

REASONS FOR CAPITAL EXPENDITURE REQUESTS

Requests for capital expenditures are usually originated by the department manager, because this individual is logistically situated in a responsibility position and hence is able to recognize the need for the capital expenditure and its impact, both economically and socially, on the department.

Depending on the health care institution involved, capital investment proposals can begin for a variety of reasons. For the purposes of analysis, capital projects may be classified into one of six categories:

1. replacement
2. improved productivity
3. improved quality of service
4. required for accreditation
5. new service
6. others

Replacement of capital equipment is usually made when the cost of repairs and maintenance exceeds the provision for depreciation or when the equipment has been totally depreciated. In some cases, the equipment just does not live up to expectations. When this occurs, it may prove best to cut the loss on the initial investment and replace the equipment.

Occasionally, similar equipment which costs approximately the same and which can improve productivity and capacity is available. In this case it may prove economically feasible to replace the present equipment with the newer model in order to improve the department's productivity.

Improved quality of the service or product generated must always be one of the goals of a department manager. If a piece of equipment is available which gives a higher quality of service compared to the present system, then a cost-benefit analysis should be conducted to consider whether or not to purchase the new equipment. If the study proves that it will be very beneficial, then the decision to purchase the new equipment is almost a foregone conclusion. If the study proves that it will be economically marginal but that purchasing the equipment gives the facility a "market edge," then a managerial decision must be made as to what would be best for the institution.

Occasionally, the health care facility may be cited for some inadequacy during the institution's accreditation review. In such cases, it is mandatory to correct the cited inadequacy, even through a nonplanned acquisition, in order to obtain or retain the facility's accreditation.

Most health care facilities are constantly looking for new sources of revenue. These new revenues may be generated through the use of new resources, personnel, and capital equipment. As stated earlier, most of these types of capital expenditure carry a high risk, owing to the uncertainty of their acceptance, need, and volume of activity. It is imperative that a comprehensive justification study, similar to the one illustrated later in this chapter, should be completed for *each* new service, together with a project budget. These two documents will assist the department manager and the facility's management team in evaluating the economic feasibility of the new service.

Other reasons a health care facility might want to invest in capital expenditures include, but are not limited to, the following:

- to expand the services
- to improve safety conditions
- to increase equipment capacity
- to reduce costs
- to improve patient care
- for the sake of convenience

Another capital expenditure classification method might be based on degrees of necessity, which could be expressed using terms such as *urgent, essential, economically desirable*, and *generally desirable*.[8] The kinds of classification system are extremely numerous. The institution's budget committee, which has the responsibility for prioritizing, giving the preliminary approval, and recommending all departmental capital expenditure plans, will usually establish the request method and criteria which are best suited to the facility's needs.

ACCOUNTING FOR CAPITAL EXPENDITURES

Typically, capital expenditures, as opposed to operating expenditures, are unique, because the total investment is not included in the institution's operating budget. Only the proportionate amount of one year's amortized depreciation may be included in the operating budget. However, the total capital investment must be included in the cash flow forecast as the payments are scheduled. Conversely, the depreciation provision is included in the operating budget but is not included in the cash flow forecast. The difference is that the acquisition of capital purchases, unless leased, usually requires a substantial cash outlay, while depreciation is an accounting procedure which only makes amortization depreciation provision over the useful life of the capital asset. Depreciation ''expense'' is a noncash transaction.

The cost of leased capital expenditures is recorded as an operating expenditure in the operating statement and as a cash outflow in the cash flow statement as the expense is incurred. No provision for depreciation is required for leased equipment.

COSTS USED TO EVALUATE CAPITAL REQUESTS

Before reviewing the mathematical methods available for evaluating capital expenditure requests, it is important to become acquainted with the following types of costs, all of which need to be considered: (1) operating costs, (2) opportunity costs, and (3) social costs.

Operating costs are the actual expenses incurred by a department in generating patient services and other functions required by the department. Operating costs include direct expenses, i.e., salaries, wages, fringe benefits, supplies, provisions for depreciation, and other related costs. Under the budgetary planning and control system, operating expenses are divided into direct and indirect costs. The budgetary process is concerned with only the direct expenses that are controllable by the department manager.

Opportunity costs are the earnings lost by the organization when the use of its services, products, or facilities is not realized from a possible capital investment because investment was instead made in an alternative use.[9]

To illustrate opportunity costs, suppose that the alternatives under consideration are identified as choices A-1, A-2, A-3, and A-4, and the related revenues and costs are as displayed in Table 5-1.

According to this analysis, alternative A-4 offers the most rewarding opportunity for Hometown Memorial Hospital, because it is forecasted to result in net earnings of $70,000. However, assume that management chose alternative A-3. In this case, the opportunity cost (OC) to the hospital would be $25,000. The OC is simply the earnings to be realized from the best opportunity (BO) minus the earnings to be realized from the selected opportunity (SO), or

$$OC = BO - SO$$

or

$$OC = \$70,000 - \$45,000$$

or

$$OC = \$25,000$$

Theoretically, health care managers accept projects which yield the greatest amount of earnings over their real operating expenditures because these contribute more to the institution. However, all knowledgeable and appropriate capital expenditure decisions need more than financial information only. By selecting A-3, perhaps management envisioned long-term benefits (e.g., improved public relations) that would more than compensate for the lesser short-term earnings given that A-4 was not chosen. Since such costs represent foregone revenues and expenses, opportunity costs are not customarily included in the general accounting system of a health care institution, but they can and should influence the investment decision.

Social costs are those costs which management knowingly or unknowingly imposes on society as a result of its decisions. For example, suppose that a health care institution's management installs a new sewage system which drains directly

---

Table 5-1 Alternative Investments for Satellite Clinic of the Emergency Services Department as of January 31, 19x2

Description	(thousands of dollars)			
	A-1	A-2	A-3	A-4
Net revenue	$360	$320	$450	$400
Relevant costs				
Inventory and site preparation	110	110	110	110
Labor and overhead	280	210	295	220
Total investment	$390	$320	$405	$330
Net earnings (loss)	$(30)	$ 0	$ 45	$ 70

into a river. This new system is a health and environmental hazard and will eventually require a major cleanup campaign. The related costs of this cleanup would be classified as social costs, regardless of who ultimately pays for the campaign.[10] Occasionally, the best alternative from the opportunity cost standpoint may have long-term social costs. Perhaps A-3 was selected over A-4 because of the latter's social costs.

In summary, opportunity costs are relatively easy to identify while social costs tend to be more difficult. Each of these types of costs must be considered, together with operating costs, when making capital investment decisions, but unfortunately most capital investment evaluation models only consider operating costs. It is important to note that the evaluation models in this text only take into account the initial investment and its related operating revenues and expenses.

MATHEMATICAL METHODS TO EVALUATE CAPITAL REQUESTS

Conceptually, the discounted cash flow analysis is superior to most mathematical evaluation models, but even this method must be used with common sense when evaluating a capital investment request. Before we examine this method, the "payback" and "bailout" payback systems will be reviewed.

Assume that Hometown Memorial Hospital's laboratory department manager submits a request for capital investment (I) of $379,000 and that the investment is expected to generate a net profit or earnings (E) of $100,000 per year. The payback period (P) required to recover the original investment would be computed as follows:

$$\frac{I}{E} = P$$

or

$$\frac{\$379,000}{\$100,000} = P$$

or

$$3.79 = P$$

The payback period is 3.79 years. In the payback model, as with most other types of capital investment evaluation models, time is the prime consideration.

The bailout system brings an additional dimension to the payback model by taking into account the salvage value of the capital investment. Using the initial information, assume that the salvage value of the investment is $250,000 at the end of the first year and that this amount declines at the rate of $50,000 per year thereafter. The bailout payback analysis is illustrated in Table 5-2.

Table 5-2 Bailout Payback Analysis of Laboratory Capital Request as of January 31, 19x2

Original investment: $379,000
First year's salvage value: $100,000
Annual decline value: $50,000

Year	Cumulative Earnings (at end of year)	+	Salvage Value	=	Cumulative Total Value
19x2	$100,000	+	$250,000	=	$350,000
19x3	200,000	+	200,000	=	400,000
19x4	300,000	+	150,000	=	450,000
19x5	400,000	+	100,000	=	500,000
19x6	500,000	+	50,000	=	550,000
19x7	600,000	+	none		600,000

The cumulative total value at the end of year 19x3 is $400,000, or more than the original investment of $379,000. Therefore, the Hometown Memorial Hospital could "bailout" of the investment at the end of the project's second complete year and not experience a financial loss. In fact, at anytime after this period, the capital investment may be totally scrapped and the investors will have recovered their original investment (except for one thing: the cost of money).

The discounted cash flow model recognizes not only the time element, but also that the use of money has a cost, just as the use of equipment has a cost (rent or lease). All things being equal, the discounted cash flow approach to evaluating capital investments considers that during an inflationary economy, a dollar has more value or worth in the present year than it will have in the future. Again using the initial laboratory capital request as an example, an application of the discounted cash flow methodology follows.

Let the original investment be $379,000, the useful life be five years, the annual estimated earnings be $100,000, and the desired rate of return be 8 percent. The desired rate of return is an arbitrary percentage which management believes the organization should realize due to present economic circumstances, e.g., the prime interest rate, inflation rate, mortgage rates, etc. Using the net present value table in Table 5-3, the discounted cash flow of this capital request can be calculated (see Table 5-4).

The laboratory capital request as computed in the worksheet in Table 5-4 produces an additional return of $20,300 or a positive net present value (+ NPV). Had the institution's management desired a rate of return larger than the identified 8 percent, the original capital investment would not have been recovered over the estimated useful life of the equipment.

Table 5-3 Present Value Table of $1.00

$$P = \frac{S}{(1 + r)^n}$$

Periods	4%	6%	8%	10%	12%	14%	16%	18%	20%	22%	24%	26%	28%	30%	40%
1	0.962	0.943	0.926	0.909	0.893	0.877	0.862	0.847	0.833	0.820	0.806	0.794	0.781	0.769	0.714
2	0.925	0.890	0.857	0.826	0.797	0.769	0.743	0.718	0.694	0.672	0.650	0.630	0.610	0.592	0.510
3	0.889	0.840	0.794	0.751	0.712	0.675	0.641	0.609	0.579	0.551	0.524	0.500	0.477	0.455	0.364
4	0.855	0.792	0.735	0.683	0.636	0.592	0.552	0.516	0.482	0.451	0.423	0.397	0.373	0.350	0.260
5	0.822	0.747	0.681	0.621	0.567	0.519	0.476	0.437	0.402	0.370	0.341	0.315	0.291	0.260	0.186
6	0.790	0.705	0.630	0.564	0.507	0.456	0.410	0.370	0.335	0.303	0.275	0.250	0.227	0.207	0.133
7	0.760	0.665	0.583	0.513	0.452	0.400	0.354	0.314	0.279	0.249	0.222	0.198	0.178	0.159	0.095
8	0.731	0.627	0.540	0.467	0.404	0.351	0.305	0.266	0.233	0.204	0.179	0.157	0.139	0.123	0.068
9	0.703	0.592	0.500	0.424	0.361	0.308	0.263	0.225	0.194	0.167	0.144	0.125	0.108	0.094	0.048
10	0.676	0.558	0.463	0.386	0.322	0.270	0.227	0.191	0.162	0.137	0.116	0.099	0.085	0.073	0.035
11	0.650	0.527	0.429	0.350	0.287	0.237	0.195	0.162	0.135	0.112	0.094	0.079	0.066	0.056	0.025
12	0.625	0.497	0.397	0.319	0.257	0.208	0.168	0.137	0.112	0.092	0.076	0.062	0.052	0.043	0.018
13	0.601	0.469	0.368	0.290	0.229	0.182	0.145	0.116	0.093	0.076	0.061	0.050	0.040	0.033	0.013
14	0.577	0.442	0.340	0.263	0.205	0.160	0.125	0.099	0.078	0.062	0.049	0.039	0.032	0.025	0.009
15	0.555	0.417	0.315	0.239	0.183	0.140	0.108	0.084	0.065	0.051	0.040	0.031	0.025	0.020	0.006
16	0.534	0.394	0.292	0.218	0.163	0.123	0.093	0.071	0.054	0.042	0.032	0.025	0.019	0.015	0.005
17	0.513	0.371	0.270	0.198	0.146	0.108	0.080	0.060	0.045	0.034	0.026	0.020	0.015	0.012	0.003
18	0.494	0.350	0.250	0.180	0.130	0.095	0.069	0.051	0.038	0.028	0.021	0.016	0.012	0.009	0.002
19	0.475	0.331	0.232	0.164	0.116	0.083	0.060	0.043	0.031	0.023	0.017	0.012	0.009	0.007	0.002
20	0.456	0.312	0.215	0.149	0.104	0.073	0.051	0.037	0.026	0.019	0.014	0.010	0.007	0.005	0.001
21	0.439	0.294	0.199	0.135	0.093	0.064	0.044	0.031	0.022	0.015	0.011	0.008	0.006	0.004	0.001
22	0.422	0.278	0.184	0.123	0.083	0.056	0.038	0.026	0.018	0.013	0.009	0.006	0.004	0.003	0.001
23	0.406	0.262	0.170	0.112	0.074	0.049	0.033	0.022	0.015	0.010	0.007	0.005	0.003	0.002	
24	0.390	0.247	0.158	0.102	0.066	0.043	0.028	0.019	0.013	0.008	0.006	0.004	0.003	0.002	
25	0.375	0.233	0.146	0.092	0.059	0.038	0.024	0.016	0.010	0.007	0.005	0.003	0.002	0.001	
26	0.361	0.220	0.135	0.084	0.053	0.033	0.021	0.014	0.009	0.006	0.004	0.002	0.002	0.001	
27	0.347	0.207	0.125	0.076	0.047	0.029	0.018	0.011	0.007	0.005	0.003	0.002	0.001	0.001	
28	0.333	0.196	0.118	0.069	0.042	0.026	0.016	0.010	0.006	0.004	0.002	0.002	0.001	0.001	
29	0.321	0.185	0.107	0.063	0.037	0.022	0.014	0.003	0.005	0.003	0.002	0.001	0.001		
30	0.308	0.174	0.099	0.057	0.033	0.020	0.012	0.007	0.004	0.003	0.002	0.001	0.001		
40	0.208	0.097	0.045	0.022	0.011	0.005	0.003	0.001	0.001						

Source: Charles T. Horngren and George Foster, *Cost Accounting: A Managerial Emphasis*, 6th ed., © 1987, p. 948. Adapted by permission of Prentice-Hall, Inc., Englewood Cliffs, N.J.

Table 5-4 Net Present Value Analysis of Laboratory Capital Request as of January 31, 19x2

Original investment: $379,000
Useful life: 5 years
Estimated annual earnings: $100,000
Desired rate of return: 8%

Year	Present Value of $1.00 at 8%	Present Value	Accumulated Value	Earnings (in thousands of dollars) 1	2	3	4	5
19x2	$ .926	$ 92,600	$ 92,600	$100				
19x3	.857	85,700	178,300		$100			
19x4	.794	79,400	257,700			$100		
19x5	.735	73,500	331,200				$100	
19x6	.681	68,100	399,300					$100
Total		$399,300		$100	$100	$100	$100	$100
Total investment		379,000						
Net return		$ 20,300						

SELECTION OF APPROPRIATE CAPITAL REQUEST

After sufficient research has been done into the types of capital investments to be considered and preliminary mathematical studies have been completed, the department manager chooses one of four alternatives before filing a formal capital expenditure request for the investment.

1. Do nothing. Either do not furnish the new service or allow the present capital equipment to deteriorate gradually and ultimately to break down.
2. Replace the present capital equipment with comparable equipment.
3. Replace the present capital equipment with lower capacity equipment.
4. Replace the present equipment with higher capacity equipment.

Each of these alternatives will have a direct impact on the department's productivity and profitability.

1. If the decision is to do nothing, the following might occur:
   - events
     —gradual increase in equipment repairs
     —eventual total equipment breakdown
   - results
     —decreased productivity
     —eventual total loss in productivity

2. If the decision is to replace the equipment with comparable equipment, the following might occur:

   - events
     —productivity remains basically the same
     —possible undercapacity to meet future demands for services
   - results
     —no increase in profit margin
     —no increase in productivity

3. If the decision is to replace the equipment with smaller capacity equipment, the following might occur:

   - events
     —processing system about the same
     —undercapacity to meet the demand
   - results
     —possible decrease in profits and lower sales
     —lower productivity

4. If the selection is to purchase equipment with higher capacity, the following might occur:

   - events
     —increased productivity
     —capacity to accommodate future demands
   - results
     —possible lower cost per production unit
     —potential greater profitability
     —possible underutilization of capacity

To summarize, a capital expenditure investment must never be made with only one alternative, one cost estimate, or one vendor's proposal. Without the opportunity to compare alternatives, the decision maker(s) will have no basis for evaluating and weighing the options and cannot make an appropriate decision.

FORMALIZING THE CAPITAL REQUEST

After the department manager has selected the capital expenditure(s) to be proposed to the budget committee, a formal request may be made in two different ways: by using (1) a consolidated departmental request or (2) an individual project request.

A consolidated departmental request (see Exhibit 5-1) lists *all* of the capital expenditure requests on one consolidated form and identifies only the key consid-

Exhibit 5-1 Consolidated Departmental Request Form

Hometown Memorial Hospital
Hometown, U.S.A.

page 1 of ____

Departmental Request for Capital Expenditures
for the Budget Year 19___

Department: _____

Department Manager: _____

Report Date: _____ 19___

Capital Expenditure		Reason for Request	Type of Asset*					Vendor	Quantity	Cost		Monthly Schedule of Acquisition											
No.	Description		L	LI	B	FE	MM			Each	Total	Jan	Feb	Mar	Apr	May	Jun	Jul	Aug	Sep	Oct	Nov	Dec

*L = Land, LI = Land Improvement, B = Building, FE = Fixed Equipment, MM = Major Movable Equipment

Exhibit 5-2 Individual Project Request Form

Hometown Memorial Hospital
Hometown, U.S.A.

page 1 of 4

Project Opportunity Package
Request for Capital Expenditure
for the Budget Year 19___

Department: _____
Department Manager: _____ Report Date: _____ 19___
Project No.: _____ Project Name: _____

1. Describe project:

2. Describe potential market:

3. Identify project competition:

4. Identify alternatives to project:

5. Describe advantages of acquiring capital asset:

6. Describe consequences if organization does not acquire capital asset:

7. Summary operating statement:

Description		*Financial Projections*	
Personnel	*Budget Year*	*Year Two*	*Year Three*
_____	$_____	$_____	$_____
_____	_____	_____	_____
Supplies			
_____	_____	_____	_____
_____	_____	_____	_____
Depreciation	_____	_____	_____
Total expenses	$_____	$_____	$_____
Net revenues	$_____	$_____	$_____
Profit (loss)	$_____	$_____	$_____

Exhibit 5-2 continued

Production unit (describe): _____

Volume of units	_____	_____	_____
Unit selling price	$_____	$_____	$_____
Unit expense	_____	_____	_____
Unit profit (loss)	$_____	$_____	$_____

8. Equipment (describe):

   Equipment bids:
   Vendor 1: _____ $_____
   Vendor 2: _____ $_____
   Vendor 3: _____ $_____

   Proposed method of acquisition:

   _____

9. Mathematical justifications:
   a. Payback method: b. Bailout method:

   c. Discounted cash flow method:

10. Break-even analysis:
    a. Fixed expenses/unit contribution ($) = B-E units

    b. Fixed expenses/unit contribution margin (%) = B-E sales

_____

Comments:

_____

Budget committee decisions:

1. _____ Finance immediately
2. _____ Defer acquisition
3. _____ Reject

Committee comments:

Decision Date: _____ 19___

Approved by: _____ Title: _____

erations concerning each. An individual project opportunity package (POP) request (see Exhibit 5-2) identifies only one capital expenditure and develops an extensive cost-benefit analysis of many key considerations and justifications (e.g., payback, earnings, etc.) to support the project.

There are as many types of capital expenditure request forms as there are health care facilities. Each organization must design the forms and request methodologies required to accommodate its particular needs. The forms displayed in this text are presented only as models for guiding institutions in designing their own forms. Remember that the form design is not as important as the information it contains or how the information is used to determine the correctness of a capital investment.[11]

NOTES

1. Allen G. Herkimer, Jr., *Understanding Hospital Financial Management,* 2d ed. (Rockville, Md.: Aspen, 1986), 263.

2. James C. Van Horne, *Financial Management and Policy* (Englewood Cliffs, N.J.: Prentice-Hall, 1971), 10.

3. Ibid., 45–46.

4. L. Vann Seawell, *Hospital Financial Accounting Theory and Practice* (Oak Brook, Ill.: Healthcare Financial Management Association, 1975), 553.

5. Ibid., 384.

6. Ibid.

7. Ibid.

8. Truman H. Esmond, Jr., *Budgeting Procedures for Hospital* (Chicago: American Hospital Publishing, 1982), 116.

9. Herkimer, *Understanding Hospital Financial Management,* 46–47.

10. Ibid., 47.

11. Ibid., 290–300.

Preliminary Revenue Budget

6

After the capital acquisitions have been identified and the volumes of activity for both the established and new services have been forecast, the next step is to generate a preliminary revenue budget based on the existing pricing structure. There are two reasons for initially projecting the revenue budget by using the existing pricing mechanisms.

First, this pricing structure represents known facts. However, if there are managed contracts (e.g., HMO, PPO, etc.) whose new rates have been received or if the health care institution has received the adjusted diagnosis related group (DRG) rate, these new rates should be used in the preliminary revenue budget.

Second, the use of the existing rate structure for the preliminary forecast assists management in maintaining a competitive price structure for its nonnegotiated rates. If after the preliminary revenue budget is completed, the net operating results are not achieved, then appropriate adjustments must be made. This process is discussed in Chapter 10. It is, however, important to remember that in order to maintain the competitive edge, raising prices must be done only as the last resort.

CLASSIFICATION OF REVENUES

Revenues are generated from the sale of goods and the rendering of services, and they are measured by the charge (price) made to the patients, clients, or tenants for goods and services furnished to them. Revenues may also include gains from the sale or exchange of assets, interest and dividends earned on investments, and unrestricted donations of resources to the health care institution.[1]

There are two important kinds of classification regarding revenues.

First, most health care institutions classify revenues as either *gross revenues* or *net revenues*.

Gross revenues represent the total amount generated for services or goods purchased by the patient or client at the "listed or published price," i.e., before any discounts have been granted to the customer. For example, assume that a patient comes into Hometown Memorial Hospital's emergency services department and the total charge for all services rendered and for supplies amounts to $175. This $175 is the gross revenue for that occasion of service.

Net revenues represent the residual from the gross revenues after the discounts have been deducted from the total. In other words, net revenues represent the maximum cash which the institution can expect to receive from the occasion of service. Assume, for example, that the emergency room patient had a Blue Cross contract. Assume further that the facility had a contractual agreement with Blue Cross stating that it would pay only 80 percent of the gross charge, of which the patient is responsible for the first $25. The balance, or 20 percent of the charge or price, would be considered as a contractual discount or allowance, as illustrated:

Gross revenue (price)		$175.00
Due from patient	25.00	
Due from Blue Cross	115.00	
Net revenue (80%)		140.00
Deduction from gross revenue		$ 35.00

In this example, the net revenue of $140 is the maximum amount of cash the facility can expect to receive from this transaction. The balance of $35 is considered as a contractual allowance without recourse to the patient.

Second, most health care institutions classify revenues as either *operating/patient care revenues* or *nonoperating/patient care revenues*. Operating/patient care revenues are generated from patient care and from health care services. Nonoperating revenues represent all revenues generated from non-patient-related sales or services, e.g., interest earned, rents, vending machine intake, sales of assets, etc. Usually, nonoperating revenues are reported at the bottom of the operating statement and "netted out" by deducting any related non-operating expenses, e.g., broker's commission, etc. For example:

Gross patient revenue	$6,500,000
Less deductions	1,500,000
Net patient revenue	$5,000,000
Less operating expenses	5,150,000
Net operating profit (loss)	$ (150,000)
Nonoperating revenue	250,000
Less nonoperating expenses	25,000
Net nonoperating revenue	$ 225,000
Net profit (loss)	$ 75,000

At first glance, it might appear that the health care facility is operating profitably. After further examination, however, the separation of the operating and the nonoperating results identifies a $150,000 loss from patient operations, which is offset by a profit of $225,000 from nonpatient operations.

These and other types of revenue classifications assist management in analyzing its operating results. The degree of revenue segmentation is dependent on management's needs.

DEDUCTIONS FROM GROSS REVENUE

As discussed previously, deductions from gross revenue represent the difference between the gross price of the health care service and the net revenue (cash) received for rendering the service. These deductions are usually separated into two major categories: *allowances* and *bad debts*.

Allowances are further segmented into *contractual allowances, courtesy allowances,* and *free work* or *charity allowances*.

A contractual allowance is the net difference, either positive or negative, between the facility's published price and the amount received from some prearranged contract or agreement with a third party payer, e.g., Blue Cross, Medicare, Medicaid, HMOs, etc. In the case of any contractual allowance, the facility has no recourse to the patient for collecting the difference between the gross or selling price and the net cash received from the third party payer. The contractual allowance is a cost of doing business.

Courtesy allowances are approved only through the governing board's policies or by an administrative policy, not through contracts. These types of allowances (e.g., employee allowances, physician allowances, etc.) may be expressed as a percentage of the gross amount of the debt, as a fixed dollar amount, or by some other arrangement documented in the facility's policies.

Free work or charity allowances represent those accounts that are to be reduced and that have been classified as such either prior to admission or at time of admission to the facility, unlike the other two kinds of allowance. "Non-Compensated Care" is another term that is commonly used to refer to this type of service. These types of deductions, which are usually based on the patient's ability to pay, can range from a minimal or partial allowance to a 100 percent write-off. These allowances are generally determined according to the health care institution's policies.

A bad debt is defined as a receivable which, despite the patient's ability to pay, is regarded as uncollectible.[2] Unlike other traditional business accounting procedures, the health care accounting and budgeting process usually requires the provision of bad debts to be recorded as a deduction from gross revenue rather than as an operating expense. Net provision for bad debts, which is the balance of the gross provision for bad debts less all amounts collected during the accounting period from previously written off bad debts, is computed as follows:

Gross provision for bad debts	$175,000
Less recoveries from bad debts	50,000
Net provision for bad debts	$125,000

Deductions from gross revenues are generally included in a department's preliminary revenue budget. Rather, most health care institutions gather all the departmental gross revenue budgets together and develop an institutional percentage for deductions from gross revenues, computed as follows:

Description	Amount	Percent
Gross revenues	$12,356,750	100%
Less deductions	2,100,648	17
Net revenues	$10,256,102	83%

Most health care institutions do not distribute a provision for deductions from gross revenues directly to each revenue-producing department, because it is virtually impossible to identify for each third party payer's accounts the proportionate amount of deductions given to each contributing department.

Since one of the purposes of our budget study is to compute a revenue department's contribution to the total institution, it is imperative that a provision for deduction from gross revenue be included in the department's revenue budget. In this study, the institutional percentage of gross revenues (in the example above, 17 percent) will be used to calculate the departmental deductions from gross revenues.

USE OF REVENUE STANDARD RATES

In a simple two-party environment, where the customer agrees to purchase a product for a specific amount, the producer would keep a record of the number of units sold annually. In order to generate a revenue budget, the producer would then multiply the total number of units, plus any anticipated increase, by the average price of the product. In this way a revenue budget could be generated. For example:

Number of units (previous year)	25,000
Plus anticipated increase	2,500
Total number of units (budget year)	27,500

This simplistic approach is not possible in most health care institutions because of the vast assortment of payers and their respective price arrangements. However, as stated in Chapter 4, our budget study is going to take the simplistic approach and consider only three types of nursing services and their respective standard revenue rates:

Type of Service	Standard Rate per Patient Day
1-bed nursing service	$350
2-bed nursing service	275
4-bed nursing service	175

The following example illustrates how January's preliminary (gross) revenue budget is generated using the standard rate for each type of service and the January patient day volumes (as projected in Table 4-9):

Type of Service	Rate	Patient Days	Gross Revenues
1-bed nursing service	$350	705	$ 246,750
2-bed nursing service	275	2,881	792,275
4-bed nursing service	175	1,354	236,950
Total		4,940	$1,275,975

SPREADSHEET APPLICATION

To apply the preliminary revenue budget process to the spreadsheet, plot the above patient days in the January column and record the appropriate gross revenues in the January gross revenue rows. Continue, in the same manner, to plot the remaining months' patient days from Table 6-1 on the four volume rows in Exhibit 6-1, and calculate the monthly gross revenue by multiplying the patient day volume by the corresponding standard rates, as illustrated in Exhibit 6-1.

Table 6-1 Medical and Surgical Patient Day Forecast by Accommodation for the Budget Year ending December 31, 19x6

Month	1-Bed	2-Bed	4-Bed	Total
January	705	2,881	1,354	4,940
February	630	2,576	1,210	4,416
March	666	2,716	1,280	4,662
April	675	2,772	1,296	4,743
May	666	2,732	1,280	4,678
June	630	2,576	1,210	4,416
July	604	2,487	1,161	4,252
August	643	2,639	1,235	4,517
September	675	2,772	1,296	4,743
October	721	2,965	1,384	5,070
November	698	2,852	1,339	4,889
December	651	2,678	1,250	4,579
Total	7,964	32,646	15,295	55,905

Exhibit 6-1 Preliminary Revenue Departmental Variable Budget for the Year Ending 31 December 19x8

Hometown Memorial Hospital
Hometown, U.S.A.

Preliminary Revenue
Departmental Variable Budget
for the Year Ending December 31, 19x8

Department: Medical & Surgical Routine Nursing

Account Number	Description	Standard Rate	January	February	March	April	May
Volume							
	1-bed patient days		705	630	666	675	666
	2-bed patient days		2881	2576	2716	2772	2732
	4-bed patient days		1354	1210	1280	1296	1280
	Total patient days		4940	4416	4662	4743	4678
Gross Revenue							
3541.01	1-bed nursing service	$350.00	$246750.00	$220500.00	$233100.00	$236250.00	$233100.00
3541.02	2-bed nursing service	$275.00	$792275.00	$708400.00	$746900.00	$762300.00	$751300.00
3541.03	4-bed nursing service	$175.00	$236950.00	$211750.00	$224000.00	$226800.00	$224000.00
	Total gross revenue		$1275975.00	$1140650.00	$1204000.00	$1225350.00	$1208400.00
Deductions from Gross Revenue							
4541.01	Medicare allowances						
4541.02	Medicaid allowances						
4541.03	Blue Cross allowances						
4541.04	Other contract allowances						
4531.05	Free work and charity						
4541.10	Bad debts						
	Total deductions	0.17	$216915.75	$193910.50	$204680.00	$208309.50	$205428.00
Net Revenue			$1059059.25	$946739.50	$999320.00	$1017040.50	$1002972.00

An institutional average deduction from gross revenue of 17 percent is used in Exhibit 6-1 to calculate the department's net revenue. For example, the department's total revenue summary is as follows:

Gross patient revenue	$14,718,350.00
Less deductions	2,502,119.50
Net patient revenue	$12,216,230.50

Although the cents amount is included in the above example, the amounts recorded in most budgets are usually carried to the nearest dollar. In some cases totals are carried to the nearest hundred or thousands of dollars depending on the size (amount) of the budget.

June	July	August	September	October	November	December	Total
630	604	643	675	721	698	651	7964
2576	2487	2639	2772	2965	2852	2678	32646
1210	1161	1235	1296	1384	1339	1250	15295
4416	4252	4517	4743	5070	4889	4579	55905
$220500.00	$211400.00	$225050.00	$236250.00	$252350.00	$244300.00	$227850.00	$2787400.00
$708400.00	$683925.00	$725725.00	$762300.00	$815375.00	$784300.00	$736450.00	$8977650.00
$211750.00	$203175.00	$216125.00	$226800.00	$518875.00	$234325.00	$218750.00	$2953300.00
$1140650.00	$1098500.00	$1166900.00	$1225350.00	$1586600.00	$1262925.00	$1183050.00	$14718350.00
$193910.50	$186745.00	$198373.00	$208309.50	$269722.00	$214697.25	$201118.50	$2502119.50
$946739.50	$911755.00	$968527.00	$1017040.50	$1316878.00	$1048227.75	$981931.50	$12216230.50

One word of caution: In any real-life situation, it is imperative that the health care institution concurrently collect, for each third party payer, comprehensive information concerning

- rates, e.g., per diem, per case, per capita rates
- production units, e.g., patient days, cases, net revenues, net expenses, etc.
- deductions from gross revenues by contract

This information, together with other relevant contractual information, is necessary in order to generate the institution's revenue budget.

To summarize, the departmental preliminary revenue budget (in our case study) has been generated using only two basic data sources: (1) the volume forecast and (2) the price per production unit.

The annual volume forecast has been distributed every month based on the present and/or the previous year's actual experience. Since this volume forecast represents management's most knowledgeable and reasonable estimate, it is not expected to change throughout the balance of the budget process. On the other hand, the second data base, which is grounded on the present price structure, may be adjusted during the sensitivity testing process in order to achieve management's desired profit margin.

NOTES

1. L. Vann Seawell, *Hospital Financial Accounting Theory and Practice* (Oak Brook, Ill.: Healthcare Financial Management Association, 1975), 556.

2. Ibid., 548.

Salary and Wage Budget

7

The health care industry has been categorized as labor-intensive. This means that the industry's major share of operating expenses arises from the use or abuse of the labor force—human resources. Depending on the facility or the department being analyzed, labor costs may range from 30 to 60 percent of the total operating expenses. One CEO is quoted as saying, ''As long as the labor cost is controlled the rest of the costs can take care of themselves . . . and we'll still make a profit.'' In essence, the CEO was implying that labor costs must be kept in appropriate proportion to the volume of the production units.

The expense budget methodology used in this text divides the health care facility's operating expenses into the following two major expense classifications and their subsections:

1. salaries and wages
   - fixed salaries and wages
   - variable salaries and wages
   - employee fringe benefits
2. non-salary-and-wage expenses
   - fixed non-salary-and-wage expenses
   - variable non-salary-and-wage expenses

The initial separation of the expense budget into these two major classifications allows the department manager to concentrate on the management and control of one type of expense at a time, e.g., labor, supplies, etc. The secondary segmentation, based on like cost behavior characteristics (i.e., fixed or variable), clusters the related expenses into manageable groups, with each group requiring different managerial approaches to planning and control.

This chapter concentrates on developing a salary and wage budget; the next is concerned with the development of the non-salary-and-wage budget. Both budgets, however, calculate their financial requirements based on the facility's (1) *production volume* and (2) *production standard rate(s)*.

The budgeted production volume represents management's best estimate of the amount of activity that will probably be realized in a department and/or institution, e.g., the number of patient days per nursing station.

The budgeted production standard represents management's most knowledgeable estimate of the average revenue rate, the average expense rate, the average number of production units per person-hour, and any other average rate (standard) which will probably be realized during the budget year. Both the volume and standard rates are based on historical data and trends, which are then adjusted to compensate for future expectations, e.g., the inflation rate, etc.

As stated earlier, the main key to a successful budget program is a reasonable and knowledgeable volume forecast. Another key to success is correlating the established volume forecast to the operating expenses (staffing and supplies). The variable budget methodology described in this text uses this approach.

DEFINITION AND PURPOSE

The salary and wage budget represents management's financial forecast of the facility's employee cost, i.e., salaries, wages, and employee fringe benefits. It is important to note, however, that independent contractors (e.g., registry nurses, physicians, auditors, etc.) are not classified as employees of a health care institution. Therefore, they are not included in the institution's salary and wage budget. Rather, they are considered as "outside purchased services" and are included in the non-salary-and-wage budget. The only expense items in the salary and wage budget are the institution's own employees, who are entitled to the organization's fringe benefit package, e.g., social security, retirement, compensation, etc.

EXPENSE SEGMENTATION

The first step in developing a salary and wage budget is the expense classification and segmentation process. The expense segmentation methodology systematically divides the salary and wage expense groups into categories based on like cost behavior, which assists management in monitoring and controlling the related expenses. For example, once a salary and wage expense item (e.g., core nursing staff) has been classified as fixed, the department manager should not be expected to change this expense because of changes in volume of activity. However, if there is a significant change in volume over a period of time, the fixed or "core" staffing requirements may need adjustment to obtain optimal efficiency. On the other hand, a variable expense item (e.g., P.R.N. nursing) must be managed on a daily or shift-to-shift basis in order that the total expense amount be maintained at a level that is directly correlated with the volume of activity, at least to a reasonable degree.

EXPENSE CLASSIFICATION

The basic principles of cost behavior, as discussed in Chapter 2 and classified in Exhibit 2-2, identify the following salary and wage expense classifications.

Account Number	Description	Fixed Expenses	Variable Expenses
	Salaries and Wages		
5541.01	Management and supervision	X	
5541.03	Core registered nurses	X	
5541.04	Core licensed practical nurses	X	
5541.05	Core nurse aides and orderlies	X	
5541.08	P.R.N. nursing staff		X
5541.09	Ward clerks & other clerical	X	
5541.10	Employee benefits	X	

The fixed expense component of the salary and wage budget should remain basically the same throughout the year regardless of volume fluctuations. When identifying an expense as fixed, it is important that the department manager be sure that it is established at an optimal level (e.g., 80 percent occupancy) and that the expense will remain constant throughout the year. When management has "bought off" on the fixed component of the salary and wage budget, the department manager can concentrate on managing the variable salary expense portion of the budget and keeping it in direct relationship to the volume of activity.

Ideally, all expenses should be managed as "variable" so that all expenses fluctuate directly with the volume of activity. This would certainly be optimizing the salary expense. Since this is virtually impossible, the department manager should be continually evaluating the fixed expenses in an effort to reduce the fixed cost component of the budget. Achieving a reduction would in turn reduce the health care facility's break-even point. Break-even analysis is discussed in Chapter 10.

The variable salary expense component should be designed so as to enable the department manager to staff these positions as closely proportional to the volume of activity as possible. One of the keys to successful cost management is reducing the portion of the fixed expense component and managing the variable expenses so that they are relatively close to the volume of activity. After the expense items have been classified and segmented, they are listed in the description column of the variable budget spreadsheet (see Exhibit 7-1).

Exhibit 7-1 Variable Budget Spreadsheet

Hometown Memorial Hospital
Hometown, U.S.A.

Salary and Wage Expenses
Departmental Variable Budget
for Year Ending 31 December 19x6

Department: Medical and Surgical Routine Nursing

Account Number	Description	Standard Rate	January	February	March	April	May	June	July	August	September	October	November	December	Total
	Volume														
	1-bed patient days		705	630	666	675	666	630	604	643	675	721	698	651	7964
	2-bed patient days		2881	2576	2716	2772	2732	2576	2487	2639	2772	2965	2852	2678	32646
	4-bed patient days		1354	1210	1280	1296	1280	1210	1161	1235	1296	1384	1339	1250	15295
	Total patient days		4940	4416	4662	4743	4678	4416	4252	4517	4743	5070	4889	4579	55905
	Monthly calendar days		31	28	31	30	31	30	31	31	30	31	30	31	365
	Core patient days		4340	3920	4340	4200	4340	4200	4340	4340	4200	4340	4200	4340	51100
	Excess core patient days		600	496	322	542	338	216	−88	177	543	730	689	209	4774
	PRN hours required		3150	2605	1690	2850	1774	1134	−462	929	2850	3832	3319	1098	24769
	Gross Revenue														
3541.01	1-bed nursing service														
3541.02	2-bed nursing service														
3541.03	4-bed nursing service														
	Total gross revenue														
	Net Revenue														
	Variable Operating Expenses														
	Variable Salary and Wage Expenses														
5541.01	Management and supervision	$1248	$38688	$34944	$38688	$37440	$38688	$37440	$38688	$38688	$37440	$38688	$37440	$38688	$455520
5541.03	Registered nurses	$2592	$80352	$72576	$80352	$77760	$80352	$77760	$80352	$80352	$77760	$80352	$77760	$80352	$946080
5541.03	Licensed practical nurses	$1326	$41106	$37128	$41106	$39780	$41106	$39780	$41106	$41106	$39780	$41106	$39780	$41106	$483990

5541.05 Nurse aides and orderlies	$1274	$39494	$35672	$39494	$38220	$39494	$39494	$38220	$39494	$38220	$39494	$465010
5541.09 Ward clerks and others	$842	$26102	$23576	$26102	$25260	$26102	$26102	$25260	$26102	$25260	$26102	$307330
Total variable salary and wage expenses		$225742	$203896	$225742	$218460	$225742	$225742	$218460	$225742	$218460	$225742	$2657930
5541.10 Employee benefits	0.25	$56436	$50974	$56436	$54615	$56436	$56436	$54615	$56436	$54615	$56436	$664482
Total Variable Salary and Wage Expense and Fringe Benefits		$282178	$254870	$282178	$273075	$282178	$282178	$273075	$282178	$273075	$282178	$3322412

FIXED SALARY AND WAGE EXPENSES

In our case study, management and supervision, as well as the "core" nursing staff, have been classified as fixed salary and wage expenses. The core nursing staff is at the optimal staffing level that management has agreed is necessary for a predetermined level of occupancy. The monthly budgeted occupancy level (see Table 7-1) has a monthly average of 87.5 percent, with each month's average occupancy exceeding the optimal occupancy of 80 percent, except July's.

For the purpose of this study, assume that Hometown Memorial Hospital has its 175 medical and surgical beds divided into six nursing stations as follows:

Nursing Station	Number of Beds
West 2	48 (4-bed)
East 2	34 (2-bed)
West 3	34
East 3	34
West 4	12 (1-bed)
East 4	13 (1-bed)
Total	175

Assume further that the fixed or core nursing staff is designed to accommodate an average daily census calculated at 80 percent occupancy as follows:

Table 7-1 Worksheet for Computation of Patient Occupancy for the Budget Year 19x6

Month	Capacity	Budget Patient Days	Percent Occupancy
January	5425	4940	0.910599
February	4900	4416	0.901224
March	5425	4662	0.859355
April	5250	4743	0.903429
May	5425	4678	0.862304
June	5250	4416	0.841143
July	5425	4252	0.783779*
August	5425	4517	0.832627
September	5250	4743	0.903429
October	5425	5070	0.934562
November	5250	4889	0.931238
December	5425	4579	0.844055
Total	63875	55905	0.875225

*Below optimal occupancy of 80%.

Nursing Station	Bed Capacity	80% Occupancy
West 2	48	39
East 2	34	27
West 3	34	27
East 3	34	27
West 4	12	9
East 4	13	10
Total	175	139

Then assume that management desires a core nursing staff level with an average of 5.25 nursing hours per patient day. The calendar day core medical and surgical nursing staff requirement can be computed to be 736 hours (see Table 7-2). These

Table 7-2 Worksheet to Compute the Calendar Day Core Medical and Surgical Nursing Staff Requirements Based on 80 Percent Average Daily Census for the Budget Year Ending December 31, 19x6

Nursing Stations	Position Hours					
	Mgt./Sup.	R.N.s	L.P.N.s	Aides/Ords.	Clerks	Total
Day Shift						
West 2	8.0	16.0	8.0	16.0	8.0	56.0
East 2	0.0	16.0	8.0	8.0	8.0	40.0
West 3	8.0	16.0	8.0	8.0	8.0	48.0
East 3	0.0	16.0	8.0	8.0	8.0	40.0
West 4	8.0	16.0	8.0	8.0	8.0	48.0
East 4	0.0	16.0	8.0	8.0	8.0	40.0
Shift total	24.0	96.0	48.0	56.0	48.0	272.0
Evening Shift						
West 2	8.0	16.0	8.0	16.0	8.0	56.0
East 2	0.0	16.0	8.0	8.0	8.0	40.0
West 3	8.0	16.0	8.0	8.0	8.0	48.0
East 3	0.0	16.0	8.0	8.0	8.0	40.0
West 4	8.0	16.0	8.0	8.0	8.0	48.0
East 4	0.0	16.0	8.0	8.0	0.0	32.0
Shift total	24.0	96.0	48.0	56.0	40.0	264.0
Night Shift						
West 2	8.0	8.0	8.0	16.0	8.0	48.0
East 2	0.0	8.0	8.0	8.0	0.0	24.0
West 3	8.0	8.0	8.0	8.0	8.0	40.0
East 3	0.0	8.0	8.0	8.0	0.0	24.0
West 4	8.0	8.0	8.0	8.0	8.0	40.0
East 4	0.0	8.0	8.0	8.0	0.0	24.0
Shift total	24.0	48.0	48.0	56.0	24.0	200.0
Grand total	72.0	240.0	144.0	168.0	112.0	736.0

data are summarized in Table 7-3, and hourly requirements are verified by using the formulae in Exhibit 7-2.

Before establishing the average calendar day cost of the core nursing staff, the following variables must be determined by management:

1. the base or minimal occupancy level
2. standard nursing hours per patient day
3. the nursing skill-level mix
4. hourly rates per nursing position
5. shift differentials
6. fringe benefits

Table 7-3 Daily Summary of Core Staff Nursing Hour Requirements by Position for the Budget Year Ending December 31, 19x6

Position	Shift			
	Day	Evening	Night	Total
Mgr./supervisors	24.0	24.0	24.0	72.0
R.N.s	96.0	96.0	48.0	240.0
L.P.N.s	48.0	48.0	48.0	144.0
Aides/orderlies	56.0	56.0	56.0	168.0
Ward clerks	48.0	40.0	24.0	112.0
Total daily hours	272.0	264.0	200.0	736.0

Exhibit 7-2 Computation of Average Core Nursing Hours

Hometown Memorial Hospital
Hometown, U.S.A.

Computation of Average Core Nursing Hours
per Calendar Day
at 80 Percent Occupancy
for the Budget Year Ending December 31, 19x6

1. Total medical and surgical nursing beds   = 175
2. Desired core occupancy   = 80%
3. Medical and surgical core daily census   = 140
4. Core nursing hours per daily census   = 5.25
5. Total nursing hours required per calendar
   day at 80% occupancy   = 736

These variables have been incorporated into Exhibit 7-3 in order to compute the average calendar day cost of nursing care by position. They are summarized as follows:

Account Number	Description	Average Calendar Cost
5541.01	Management and supervision	$1,248.00
5541.02	Registered nurses	2,592.00
5541.03	Licensed practical nurses	1,326.00
5541.05	Aides and orderlies	1,274.00
5541.09	Ward clerks	842.80
	Total	$7,282.80

Using the variable budget spreadsheet (Exhibit 7-1), plot these average calendar day costs in the standard rate column relating to the core nursing positions. To compute the monthly core nursing staff costs, multiply the number of calendar days in the appropriate month by the standard calendar day nursing rates. For example, January's core nursing expenses would be computed as follows:

Position	Standard Rate	Calendar Days	Monthly Expense
Management and supervision	$1,248.00	31	$ 38,688.00
Registered nurses	2,592.00	31	80,352.00
Licensed practical nurses	1,326.00	31	41,106.00
Aides & orderlies	1,274.00	31	39,494.00
Ward clerks	842.80	31	26,102.00
Total			$225,742.00

To verify the total cost of the core nursing staff, multiply the daily core cost of $7,282.80 by 365 calendar days, as follows:

$$\$7,282.80 \times 365 = \$2,658,222$$
$$\text{Spreadsheet total} = \underline{2,657,930}$$
$$\text{Difference} \quad = \quad 292$$

Even though the core nursing staff is considered a fixed salary and wage expense, the calendar day standard rates are used in a similar fashion whenever a variable expense standard rate is used. The difference is that the core salary expenses are computed based on the calendar day, while variable expenses are computed based on the volume of activity.

Exhibit 7-3 Computation of Nursing Staff Costs

Hometown Memorial Hospital
Hometown, U.S.A.

Computation of Calendar Day
Core Nursing Staff Costs
at 80% Occupancy
for the Budget Year Ending December 31, 19x6

Position	Day	Evening	Night	Total	Rate	Day	Evening		Night		Total
						Base	Base	Diff.	Base	Diff.	
Management & Supervision	24	24	24	72	$16.00	$384.00	$384.00	$57.60	$384.00	$38.40	$1,248.00
Registered Nurses	96	96	48	240	10.00	960.00	960.00	144.00	480.00	48.00	2,592.00
Licensed Practical Nurses	48	48	48	144	8.50	408.00	408.00	61.20	408.00	40.80	1,326.00
Aides & Orderlies	56	56	56	168	7.00	392.00	392.00	58.80	392.00	39.20	1,274.00
Ward Clerks	48	40	24	112	7.00	336.00	280.00	42.00	168.00	16.80	842.80
Total	272	264	200	736		2,480.00	2,424.00	363.60	1,832.00	183.20	7,282.80

VARIABLE SALARY AND WAGE EXPENSES

The variable portion of salary and wage expenses (which fluctuates directly with the volume of activity) represents the additional or P.R.N. staffing required to maintain the quality of staffing at the current activity level. The monthly patient days in excess of the core staffing level of 80 percent (see Table 7-4) assist in calculating the P.R.N. nursing hours required to maintain a nursing standard of 5.25 hours per patient day.

It can be seen that July has a negative hourly requirement of 462 hours. Since management has agreed that the core staff is to remain fixed as long as patient occupancy maintains a level substantially above 80 percent, the negative 462 hours of P.R.N. time should not affect the core staff expenses. Management needs plan no additional P.R.N. nursing staff during the month of July and must make every effort to reduce subsequent P.R.N. staffing hours by 462 hours.

The P.R.N. hour requirements (calculated in Table 7-4) are plotted as a row in the variable budget spreadsheet (see Exhibit 7-1) under the heading "P.R.N. hours required" (which is under the general heading "Volume"). Assume that $9.90 is the standard hourly wage for P.R.N. staff. The monthly P.R.N. hours required are then multiplied by the standard hourly wage of $9.90 to compute the monthly cost. For example, the P.R.N. nursing staff expenses for the month of January would be computed as follows:

Table 7-4 Worksheet for the Computation of P.R.N. Nursing Staff Requirements for the Budget Year Ending December 31, 19x6

Month	Patient Day Capacity	Budgeted Patient Days	Core 80% Patient Days	Excess Patient Days	P.R.N. Hours Required*
January	5,425	4,940	4,340	600	3,150
February	4,900	4,416	3,920	496	2,605
March	5,425	4,662	4,340	322	1,690
April	5,250	4,743	4,200	542	2,850
May	5,425	4,678	4,340	338	1,774
June	5,250	4,416	4,200	216	1,134
July	5,425	4,252	4,340	(88)	(462)
August	5,425	4,517	4,340	177	929
September	5,250	4,743	4,200	543	2,850
October	5,425	5,070	4,340	730	3,832
November	5,250	4,889	4,200	689	3,319
December	5,425	4,579	4,340	209	1,098
Total	63,875	55,905	51,100	4,774	24,769

*Nursing staffing standard of 5.25 hours per patient day

Account Number	Description	Standard Hourly Rate	P.R.N. Hours Required	Total Expense
5541.08	P.R.N. nursing staff	$9.90	3,150	$31,185.00

EMPLOYEE FRINGE BENEFITS

Employee fringe benefits include but are not limited to the following:

- employee pension plans
- health insurance
- life insurance
- compensation insurance
- vacation
- sick leave
- holidays

These benefits and any others that the health care facility chooses to give its employees are frequently tied directly into an employee's salary or wage earnings. For many of these expense items, the exact cost can be specifically identified, and for these it is appropriate to budget on a line-by-line basis. In other cases, when an exact amount is impossible to identify and calculate, it is appropriate to select a percentage of the salary and wage budget as the fringe benefit cost for the institution. For the purpose of simplification, we have selected for our case study a fringe benefit standard rate of 25 percent. Refer to the variable budget spreadsheet (Exhibit 7-1) and post .25 in the standard rate column as the standard employee fringe benefit rate. For each month, multiply this amount by that month's total fixed salaries and wages to arrive at the total monthly cost of employee fringe benefits for the fixed salary and wage section. Since P.R.N.s are not entitled to any fringe benefits, no provision for variable fringe benefits is required. The fixed employee fringe benefit costs for the month of January would be computed in the variable budget spreadsheet (Exhibit 7-1) and summarized as follows:

Position	Monthly Salary Expenses	Fringe Standard Rate	Total Fringe Expenses
Management & supervision	$ 38,688.00	.25	$ 9,673.00
Registered nurses	80,352.00	.25	20,088.00
Licensed practical nurses	41,106.00	.25	10,276.00
Aides & orderlies	39,494.00	.25	9,873.00
Ward Clerks	26,102.00	.25	6,526.00
Total	$225,742.00	.25	$56,436.00

In this chapter salary and wages are classified as either fixed or variable, with full awareness that many of the variable expenses are usually handled as step- or semivariable expenses. Step-variables are not incorporated into our case study because after the optimal level of fixed expenses has been mutually agreed on by the facility's management and departments, the department managers and their supervisors are encouraged to manage the variable expenses more effectively by eliminating the step-variable component. Department managers must concentrate on lowering the fixed portion of the salary and wage budget and manage the variable expenses so that they are in direct relationship to the volume of activity.

Chapter 8

Non-Salary-and-Wage Budget

8

Non-salary-and-wage expenses are operating expenses not related to any payroll compensation paid directly to the health care facility's employees. Any labor expense for other than the facility's own employees (those for whom W-2 forms must be filed) should be categorized as either *purchased* or *contracted services* and managed as a non-salary-and-wage expense item. A 1099 form must be filed for such items when reporting to the Internal Revenue Service.

As with the salary and wage budget, the non-salary-and-wage budget has two major categories:

1. fixed non-salary-and-wage expenses
2. variable non-salary-and-wage expenses

The fixed portion of the non-salary-and-wage expenses tends to remain the same over a relevant range of activity. For example, the rent or lease of equipment will remain constant until the volume of activity becomes so great that additional space or machine capacity is needed. (See Figure 8-1, where $40,000 has been identified as the facility's fixed costs.)

A facility's total variable non-salary-and-wage expenses tend to vary in direct proportion to the facility's volume of activity, as illustrated in Figure 8-2.

The facility's non-salary-and-wage budget assumes a configuration such as that illustrated in Figure 8-3, which is generated from the data in Table 8-1.

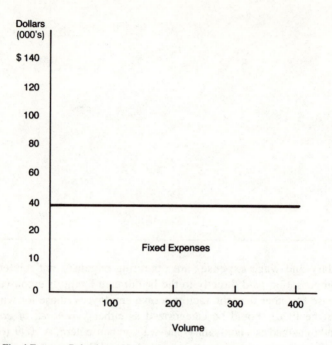

Figure 8-1 Fixed Expense Behavior at Various Levels of Activity

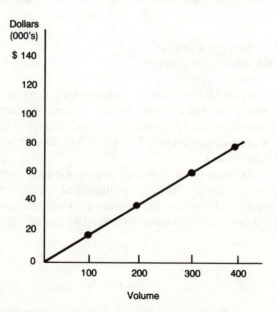

Figure 8-2 Variable Expense Behavior at Various Levels of Activity

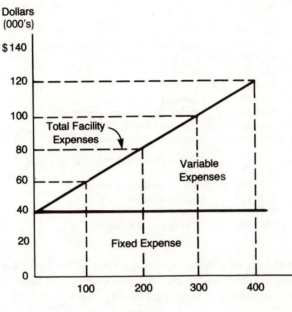

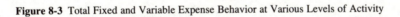

Figure 8-3 Total Fixed and Variable Expense Behavior at Various Levels of Activity

Table 8-1 Comparative Analysis of Total Facility Expenses and Average Unit Cost

Type of Expense	Volume of Activity (Units)			
	100	200	300	400
Total fixed expense	$ 40,000	$ 40,000	$ 40,000	$ 40,000
Total variable expense	20,000	40,000	60,000	80,000
Total department expense	$ 60,000	$ 80,000	$100,000	$120,000
Average cost per unit	$ 600	$ 400	$ 333	$ 300

EXPENSE CLASSIFICATION

In our case study, expense classifications which were identified for the non-salary-and-wage expense budget in Exhibit 2-2 are as follows:

Account Number	Description
	Fixed Non-Salary-and-Wage Expenses
6541.21	Dues & subscriptions
6541.25	Depreciation
6541.26	Insurance
6541.27	Equipment leases
6541.28	Training programs and conferences
6541.29	Educational travel
6541.30	Recruitment fees & expenses
	Variable Non-Salary-and-Wage Expenses
6541.15	Office supplies
6541.19	Medical and surgical supplies
6541.22	Pharmaceuticals
6541.35	Registry fees
6541.50	Other operating expenses

Referring to the variable budget spreadsheet in Exhibit 8-1, list all of the non-salary-and-wage accounts in the description column, and enter the following monthly fixed non-salary-and-wage expenses as follows:

Account Number	Description	Monthly Amount	Annual Total
6541.21	Dues & subscriptions	$ 1,000.00	$ 12,000.00
6541.25	Depreciation	22,500.00	270,000.00
6541.26	Insurance	9,500.00	114,000.00
6541.27	Equipment leases	15,400.00	184,800.00
6541.28	Training programs	3,000.00	36,000.00
6541.30	Recruitment fees & expenses	8,000.00	96,000.00

These expenses, as classified, will not significantly change each month regardless of the volume of activity. The monthly amount, therefore, should be placed in each monthly column and cross-footed to the totals.

The only identified fixed expense which is not listed is educational travel (account no. 6541.29). Although this expense has been classified as a fixed expense, it may be called a ''programmed'' expense, because it has the following unique features:

1. The annual total remains the same, or fixed, regardless of the volume of activity.
2. It is programmed to be spent disproportionately at specific times throughout the year.

Exhibit 8-1 Non-Salary-and-Wage Expenses

Hometown Memorial Hospital
Hometown, U.S.A.

Non-Salary-and-Wage Expenses
Departmental Variable Budget
for Year Ending 31 December 19x6

Department: Medical and Surgical Routine Nursing

Account Number	Description	Standard Rate	January	February	March	April	May	June	July	August	September	October	November	December	Total
	Volume														
	1-bed patient days		705	630	666	675	666	630	604	643	675	721	698	651	7964
	2-bed patient days		2881	2576	2716	2772	2732	2576	2487	2639	2772	2965	2852	2678	32646
	4-bed patient days		1354	1210	1280	1296	1280	1210	1161	1235	1296	1384	1339	1250	15295
	Total patient days		4940	4416	4662	4743	4678	4416	4252	4517	4743	5070	4889	4579	55905
	Variable Non-Salary-and-Wage Expenses														
6541.15	Office supplies	$1.50	$7410	$6624	$6993	$7114	$7017	$6624	$6378	$6775	$7114	$7605	$7333	$6868	$83857
6541.19	Medical and surgical supplies	$9.75	$48165	$43056	$45454	$46244	$45610	$43056	$41457	$44041	$46244	$49432	$47668	$44645	$545074
6541.22	Pharmaceuticals	$8.25	$40755	$36432	$38462	$39130	$38594	$36432	$35079	$37265	$39130	$41828	$40334	$37777	$461216
6541.35	Registry Fees	$15.00	$74100	$66240	$69930	$71145	$70170	$66240	$63780	$67755	$71145	$76050	$73335	$68685	$838575
6541.50	Other operating expenses	$3.75	$18525	$16560	$17482	$17786	$17542	$16560	$15945	$16939	$17786	$19012	$18334	$17171	$209644
	Total variable non-salary-and-wage expenses		$188955	$168912	$178321	$181419	$178933	$168912	$162639	$172775	$181419	$193927	$187004	$175146	$2138366
	Total Variable Operating Expenses														
	Fixed Non-Salary-and-Wage Expenses	$1000													
6541.21	Dues and subscriptions		$1000	$1000	$1000	$1000	$1000	$1000	$1000	$1000	$1000	$1000	$1000	$1000	$12000
6541.25	Depreciation		$22500	$22500	$22500	$22500	$22500	$22500	$22500	$22500	$22500	$22500	$22500	$22500	$270000
6541.26	Insurance		$9500	$9500	$9500	$9500	$9500	$9500	$9500	$9500	$9500	$9500	$9500	$9500	$114000
6541.27	Equipment leases		$15400	$15400	$15400	$15400	$15400	$15400	$15400	$15400	$15400	$15400	$15400	$15400	$184800
6541.28	Training programs		$3000	$3000	$3000	$3000	$3000	$3000	$3000	$3000	$3000	$3000	$3000	$3000	$36000
6541.29	Educational travel		$0	$0	$6000	$0	$0	$0	$0	$0	$12000	$2000	$4000	$0	$24000
6541.30	Recruitment fees, etc.		$8000	$8000	$8000	$8000	$8000	$8000	$8000	$8000	$8000	$8000	$8000	$8000	$96000
	Total fixed non-salary-and-wage expenses		$59400	$59400	$65400	$59400	$59400	$59400	$59400	$59400	$71400	$61400	$63400	$59400	$736800

For the purpose of illustration, we will assume that there are two major educational conventions to be held in March and September. Consequently, these two months receive the greatest portion of the annual expense budget and October and November receive lesser amounts, as shown:

Month	Amount
March	$ 6,000.00
September	12,000.00
October	2,000.00
November	4,000.00
Total	$24,000.00

The remaining months receive no allotment of this fixed or programmed expense category. Since programmed expenses are budgeted for specific times throughout the year, they will be provided for in the institution's cash flow forecast in the proper spending schedule. Cash flow forecasting is discussed in Chapter 9.

DEVELOPING STANDARD VARIABLE NON-SALARY-AND-WAGE RATES

As with variable salary and wage expenses, variable non-salary-and-wage expenses maintain a direct relationship between each expense item's standard rate and the monthly volume of activity. The standard variable costs (rates) used in the medical and surgical routine nursing study are as follows:

Account Number	Description	Standard Rate
6541.15	Office supplies	$ 1.50
6541.19	Medical & surgical supplies	9.75
6541.22	Pharmaceuticals	8.25
6541.35	Registry fees	15.00
6541.50	Other operating expenses	3.75

The formula used to compute the office supplies standard rate is as follows:

Let

P = previous year's actual total expense item
I = budget year's anticipated inflation rate
R = budget year's variable standard per expense item
V = budget year's anticipated volume of activity

Formula:

$$R = \frac{P + (P \times I)}{V}$$

Applying this formula, let P = $79,665, I = .0526, and V = 55,905.

$$R = \frac{\$79,665 + (\$79,665 \times .0526)}{55,905}$$

or

$$R = \frac{\$79,665 + \$4,190}{55,905}$$

or

$$R = \frac{\$83,855}{55,905}$$

or

$$R = \$1.50$$

The standard variable rate (R) for medical and surgical routine nursing office supplies (account no. 6541.15) is $1.50.

This rate may be proofed by multiplying the annual volume (55,905) by the standard rate ($1.50) and comparing the result to the amount in the total column of the variable budget spreadsheet:

55,905 × $1.50	=	$83,857.50
Spreadsheet total		83,857.50
Difference		$ 0

This formula, or an adaptation, can be applied to compute the remaining standard variable expense item rates for the rest of the standard rates.

In computing standard variable rates, the following three types of data are critical:

1. *Previous year's total item expense*. This is the actual amount spent during the previous year and is the only "hard" piece of data that can be supported by the facility's accounting department.
2. *Budget volume of activity*. This must realistically reflect management's best estimate of the number of production units the health care facility anticipates it will generate.

3. *Inflation rate*. This represents management's best estimate of the inflation rate and can be based on economic forecast projections by government or financial institutions.

It should be obvious by now that budgeting is not an exact science; it is, rather, an art. Management has the responsibility and must take the opportunity to refine the basic budgeting process during each budget year so that it becomes more automatic and the results more accurate with each iteration.

Evaluating the Preliminary Budget

9

The preliminary budget developed in our case study, illustrated in Exhibit 9-1 and summarized in Exhibit 9-2, is based on the following guidelines:

1. The volume forecast is based on management's knowledgeable and reasonable judgment.
2. The capital expenditure plan reflects what the institution realistically expects to acquire and invest. Provisions for these capital investments are included in the institution's volume forecast.
3. The revenue budget utilizes the current pricing structure of the volume forecast.
4. The expense budget is calculated (using the volume forecast) at a production rate which optimizes the facility's resources.

The most important guideline is the third, because the preliminary revenue budget is calculated at the current price structure.

Before the current rate structure is adjusted so that the institution or department can realize management's desired profit margin, the following factors must be confirmed:

1. The volume forecast is realistic and attainable.
2. The projected operating expenses generate the desired productivity level and optimize the facility's resources.
3. The planned capital investments are required to serve identified market needs and the related cost-benefit analysis meets management's desired rate of return.
4. The current pricing structure has an appropriate cost-price relationship.

135

Exhibit 9-1 Departmental Variable Detail Budget

Hometown Memorial Hospital
Hometown, U.S.A.

Departmental Variable Detail Budget
for Year Ending 31 December 19x6

Department: Medical and Surgical Routine Nursing

Account Number	Description	Standard Rate	January	February	March	April	May	June	July	August	September	October	November	December	Total
Volume															
	1-bed patient days		705	630	666	675	666	630	604	643	675	721	698	651	7964
	2-bed patient days		2881	2576	2716	2772	2732	2576	2487	2639	2772	2965	2852	2678	32646
	4-bed patient days		1354	1210	1280	1296	1280	1210	1161	1235	1296	1384	1339	1250	15295
	Total patient days		4940	4416	4662	4743	4678	4416	4252	4517	4743	5070	4889	4579	55905
	Monthly calendar days		31	28	31	30	31	30	31	31	30	31	30	31	365
	Core patient days		4340	3920	4340	4200	4340	4200	4340	4340	4200	4340	4200	4340	51100
	Excess core patient days		600	496	322	542	338	216	−88	177	543	730	689	209	4774
	PRN hours required		3150	2605	1690	2850	1774	1134	−462	929	2850	3832	3319	1098	24769
Gross Revenue															
3541.01	1-bed nursing service	$350	$246750	$220500	$233100	$236250	$233100	$220500	$211400	$225050	$236250	$252350	$244300	$227850	$2787400
3541.02	2-bed nursing service	$275	$792275	$708400	$746900	$762300	$751300	$708400	$683925	$725725	$762300	$815375	$784300	$736450	$8977650
3541.03	4-bed nursing service	$175	$236950	$211750	$224000	$226800	$224000	$211750	$203175	$216125	$226800	$518875	$234325	$218750	$2953300
	Total gross revenue		$1275975	$1140650	$1204000	$1225350	$1208400	$1140650	$1098500	$1166900	$1225350	$1586600	$1262925	$1183050	$14718350
Deductions from Gross Revenue															
4541.01	Medicare allowances														
4541.02	Medicaid allowances														
4541.03	Blue Cross allowances														
4541.04	Other contract allowances														
4531.05	Free work and charity														
4541.10	Bad debts														
	Total deductions	0.17	$216916	$193910	$204680	$208310	$205428	$193910	$186745	$198373	$208310	$269722	$214697	$201118	$2502120

Item	Rate	1	2	3	4	5	6	7	8	9	10	11	12	Total
Net Revenue		$1059059	$946740	$999320	$1017040	$1002972	$946740	$911755	$968527	$1017040	$1316878	$1048228	$981932	$12216230
Variable Operating Expenses														
Variable Salaries and Wages														
5541.03 Registered nurses														
5541.04 Licensed practical nurses														
5541.05 Nurse aides and orderlies														
5541.09 Ward clerks and others														
5541.10 Employee benefits														
5541.09 PRN nursing staff	$9.90	$31185	$25790	$16731	$28215	$17563	$11227	$0	$9197	$28215	$37937	$32858	$10870	$249788
Total variable salaries and wages		$31185	$25790	$16731	$28215	$17563	$11227	$0	$9197	$28215	$37937	$32858	$10870	$249788
Variable Non-Salary-and-Wage Expenses														
6541.15 Office supplies	$1.50	$7410	$6624	$6993	$7114	$7017	$6624	$6378	$6776	$7115	$7605	$7334	$6868	$83858
6541.19 Medical and surgical supplies	$9.75	$48165	$43056	$45454	$46244	$45610	$43056	$41457	$44041	$46244	$49432	$47668	$44645	$545074
6541.22 Pharmaceuticals	$8.25	$40755	$36432	$38462	$39130	$38594	$36432	$35079	$37265	$39130	$41828	$40334	$37777	$461216
6541.35 Registry fees	$15.00	$74100	$66240	$69930	$71145	$70170	$66240	$63780	$67755	$71145	$76050	$73335	$68685	$838575
6541.50 Other operating expenses	$3.75	$18525	$16560	$17482	$17786	$17542	$16560	$15945	$16939	$17786	$19012	$18334	$17171	$209644
Total variable non-salary-and-wage expenses		$188955	$168912	$178322	$181419	$178933	$168912	$162639	$172776	$181420	$193928	$187005	$175146	$2138367
Total Variable Operating Expenses		$220140	$194702	$195053	$209634	$196496	$180139	$162639	$181973	$209635	$231865	$219863	$186016	$2388155
Fixed Operating Expenses														
Fixed Salaries and Wages														
5541.01 Management and supervision	$1248	$38688	$34944	$38688	$37440	$38688	$37440	$38688	$38688	$37440	$38688	$37440	$38688	$455520
5541.03 Registered nurses	$2592	$80352	$72576	$80352	$77760	$80352	$77760	$80352	$80352	$77760	$80352	$77760	$80352	$946080
5541.04 Licensed practical nurses	$1326	$41106	$37128	$41106	$39780	$41106	$39780	$41106	$41106	$39780	$41106	$39780	$41106	$483990
5541.05 Nurse aides and orderlies	$1274	$39494	$35672	$39494	$38220	$39494	$38220	$39494	$39494	$38220	$39494	$38220	$39494	$465010
5541.09 Ward clerks and others	$842	$26102	$23576	$26102	$25260	$26102	$25260	$26102	$26102	$25260	$26102	$25260	$26102	$307330
Total fixed salaries and wages		$225742	$203896	$225742	$218460	$225742	$218460	$225742	$225742	$218460	$225742	$218460	$225742	$2657930
5541.10 Employee benefits	0.25	$56436	$50974	$56436	$54615	$56436	$54615	$56436	$56436	$54615	$56436	$54615	$56436	$664486
Total fixed salaries wages, and fringe benefits		$282178	$254870	$282178	$273075	$282178	$273075	$282178	$282178	$273075	$282178	$273075	$282178	$3322416

Exhibit 9-1 continued

Account Number	Description	Standard Rate	January	February	March	April	May	June	July	August	September	October	November	December	Total
	Fixed Non-Salary-and-Wage Expenses														
6541.21	Dues and subscriptions		$1000	$1000	$1000	$1000	$1000	$1000	$1000	$1000	$1000	$1000	$1000	$1000	$12000
6541.25	Depreciation		$22500	$22500	$22500	$22500	$22500	$22500	$22500	$22500	$22500	$22500	$22500	$22500	$270000
6541.26	Insurance		$9500	$9500	$9500	$9500	$9500	$9500	$9500	$9500	$9500	$9500	$9500	$9500	$114000
6541.27	Equipment leases		$15400	$15400	$15400	$15400	$15400	$15400	$15400	$15400	$15400	$15400	$15400	$15400	$184800
6541.28	Training programs		$3000	$3000	$3000	$3000	$3000	$3000	$3000	$3000	$3000	$3000	$3000	$3000	$36000
6541.29	Educational travel		$0	$0	$6000	$0	$0	$0	$0	$0	$12000	$2000	$4000	$0	$24000
6541.30	Recruitment fees, etc.		$8000	$8000	$8000	$8000	$8000	$8000	$8000	$8000	$8000	$8000	$8000	$8000	$96000
	Total fixed non-salary-and-wage expenses		$59400	$59400	$65400	$59400	$59400	$59400	$59400	$59400	$71400	$61400	$63400	$59400	$736800
	Total Fixed Operating Expenses		$341578	$314270	$347578	$332475	$341578	$332475	$341578	$341578	$344475	$343578	$336475	$341578	$4059216
	Total Fixed and Variable Expenses		$561718	$508972	$542631	$542109	$538074	$512614	$504217	$523551	$554110	$575443	$556338	$527594	$6447371
	Net Operating Contribution		$497341	$437768	$456689	$474931	$464898	$434126	$407538	$444976	$462930	$741435	$491890	$454338	$5768859

Exhibit 9-2 Departmental Summary Budget

Hometown Memorial Hospital
Hometown, U.S.A.

Medical and Surgical Routine Nursing Services
Departmental Summary Budget
for the Year Ending December 31, 19x6

Description	Amount	Percent
Volume		
Patient days	55,905	NA
Revenue		
Gross revenue	$14,718,350	100.00%
Less deductions from gross revenue	2,502,120	17.00
Net revenue	$12,216,230	83.00
Expenses		
Fixed salary and wage expenses	$3,322,416	22.57
Fixed non-salary-and-wage expenses	736,800	5.01
Total fixed expenses	$4,059,216	27.58
Variable salary and wage expenses	$ 249,788	1.70
Variable non-salary-and-wage expenses	2,138,366	14.53
Total variable expenses	$2,388,157	16.23
Total fixed and variable expenses	$6,447,371	43.81
Net contribution	$5,768,859	39.19

If these four factors have been verified and the revenue budget still does not generate management's desired profit margin, then and only then are prices raised and/or adjusted. The techniques in this chapter are designed to assist management in evaluating the preliminary budget.

For the purpose of the case study, assume that a minimum of 35 percent is what management expects from the medical and surgical nursing service department and that 39.19 percent is anticipated. The balance of this text is directed to Hometown Memorial Hospital's total operations.

COST-PRICE RELATIONSHIP

Traditionally, the budgeting process deals only with the direct expenses of a responsibility center. The hypothesis is that one person, the department manager, is placed in the responsibility position for one specific cost/revenue center, is held accountable for all its expenses and/or revenues, and must have the authority to control them. These budgeted expenses are classified as *controllable* or *direct expenses*. The *noncontrollable* or *indirect expenses*, sometimes referred to as *overhead expenses*, are the direct expenses of departments which render service to other centers.

In evaluating the profitability of a revenue-producing center, a provision must be made through the organization's pricing structure to recoup the indirect and direct expenses of the department. If this is not done, non-revenue-producing departments (e.g., housekeeping, plant, administration, etc.) will not have their direct expenses recovered and the institution will experience an operating loss and a cash shortfall. Therefore, the preliminary budget of each revenue-producing department, based on the existing price structure, must be analyzed for departmental profitability. If the profit level does not meet management's desires, then a revised pricing structure is in order. One process which can assist management in selecting the optimal price for the department's production units is called *sensitivity testing*. The methodology used to develop a revenue-producing department's total operating costs is called *cost finding*.

COST FINDING: DEFINITION AND PURPOSE

Cost finding is the allocation of the costs of non-revenue-producing departments to the revenue-producing departments. This process is accomplished through the use of statistical bases determined by the amount of services rendered by each department to the others.[1] The purpose of the cost finding process is to determine the true or total cost of operating the revenue-producing departments of a health care organization.[2]

Some of the objectives of cost finding in a health care facility or department are to provide information for

- determining the total cost of a revenue-producing department or facility
- determining the profitability by matching a department's total operating expenses to its total net revenue
- determining the price of a production unit of a revenue-producing department or facility
- conducting price sensitivity testing to establish optimal profits and/or competitive position
- conducting break-even analyses to assist management in risk-based contract negotiating

In summary, health care managers must know the total operating expenses of each of their revenue-producing departments and its production units so as to be able to effectively negotiate risk-based contracts for departmental and/or facility services. The key to successful contract negotiating is knowing the costs. With this information the negotiator is in the enviable position of knowing the price range within which the organization can profitably maneuver; without it, the contracting facility is at the complete mercy of the contractee. Under certain circumstances, some "planned" negative contracts can ultimately be beneficial for achieving an organization's long-range goals, but devising such contracts should never be a constant or unending practice.

COST FINDING: ITS APPLICATION IN BUDGETING

The spreadsheet (see Exhibit 9-3) is an example of the basic cost finding format which is commonly used in the health care industry. It is divided into two major sections. The first or top section lists the non-revenue-producing or administration/general service departments. Non-revenue-producing departments are generally listed with the cost center which provides the greatest amount of services to other departments but receives the least (e.g., insurance and interest) at the top. The list ends with the department which provides the least amount of services to other departments (e.g., medical education).

The second or bottom section comprises all the institution's revenue-producing departments, with the ancillary and nursing services grouped together.

The expenses of the non-revenue-producing departments are distributed to the revenue-producing centers using the statistical basis which best measures the amount of services rendered to the revenue-producing departments (e.g., pounds of laundry, meals served to patients, hours of housekeeping service, etc.). Ultimately, all of the non-revenue-producing departmental expenses are absorbed within the revenue-producing departments.

For many years, three basic methods of cost finding have been recommended by the American Hospital Association (AHA). They are often referred to simply as *method one, method two,* and *method three,* but other methods, such as simultaneous equations and similar algebraic formulae are also used. The resulting cost distribution generally differs slightly with each method. Because of its simplicity and Medicare's preference for it, the step-down method (AHA's method two) is almost universally used throughout the health care industry.[3]

The *short-formula 1* is one of the algebraic methods of cost finding.[4] It is an abbreviated approach to cost allocation based on the health care facility's most recent comprehensive cost finding report. Percentages of overhead ratios are developed (see Table 9-1) and applied to the current total actual or budgeted ex-

Exhibit 9-3 Cost Finding Worksheet

Hometown Memorial Hospital
Hometown, U.S.A.

Cost Finding Worksheet
for the Budget Year 19x6

Department	Direct Costs	Allocated Costs										Total Costs
		II	AG	HK	LL	OP	RM	NA	IR	MR	SS	
Non-Revenue-Producing Departments												
Insurance & interest	XXXXX	XX										
Admin. & general	XXXXX	XX	XX									
Housekeeping	XXXXX	XX	XX	XX								
Laundry & linen	XXXXX	XX	XX	XX	XX							
Operation of plant	XXXXX	XX	XX	XX	XX	XX						
Repairs & maintenance	XXXXX	XX	XX	XX	XX	XX	XX					
Nursing admin.	XXXXX	XX	XX	XX	XX	XX	XX	XX				
Interns & residents	XXXXX	XX	XX	XX	XX	XX	XX	XX	XX			
Medical records & QA	XXXXX	XX	XX	XX	XX	XX	XX	XX	XX	XX		
Social service	XXXXX	XX	XX	XX	XX	XX	XX	XX	XX	XX	XX	
Subtotal												
Revenue-Producing Departments												
Med & surg nursing	XXXXX	XX	XX	XX	XX	XX	XX	XX	XX	XX	XX	XXXXXX
ICU/CCU nursing	XXXXX	XX	XX	XX	XX	XX	XX	XX	XX	XX	XX	XXXXXX
Operating rooms	XXXXX	XX	XX	XX	XX	XX	XX	XX	XX	XX	XX	XXXXXX
Postoperative room	XXXXX	XX	XX	XX	XX	XX	XX	XX	XX	XX	XX	XXXXXX
Anesthesiology	XXXXX	XX	XX	XX	XX	XX	XX	XX	XX	XX	XX	XXXXXX
Radiology	XXXXX	XX	XX	XX	XX	XX	XX	XX	XX	XX	XX	XXXXXX
Pathology	XXXXX	XX	XX	XX	XX	XX	XX	XX	XX	XX	XX	XXXXXX
Physical therapy	XXXXX	XX	XX	XX	XX	XX	XX	XX	XX	XX	XX	XXXXXX
Respiratory therapy	XXXXX	XX	XX	XX	XX	XX	XX	XX	XX	XX	XX	XXXXXX
Pharmacy	XXXXX	XX	XX	XX	XX	XX	XX	XX	XX	XX	XX	XXXXXX
Emergency services	XXXXX	XX	XX	XX	XX	XX	XX	XX	XX	XX	XX	XXXXXX
Ambulatory clinic	XXXXX	XX	XX	XX	XX	XX	XX	XX	XX	XX	XX	XXXXXX
Total	XXXXXXX	XX	XX	XX	XX	XX	XX	XX	XX	XX	XX	XXXXXXX

penses of the non-revenue-producing departments and then added to the revenue-producing department's direct expenses. These departmental totals can be matched to each department's net revenue so as to compute the department's profitability (see Table 9-2).

Table 9-1 Analysis of Revenue-Producing Departmental Overhead Rates of Non-Revenue-Producing Departmental Expenses Based on the Comprehensive Cost Study for the Year Ending September 30, 19x5

	(1) Direct Expense	(2) Total Expense	(3) Indirect Expense	(4) Percent of Overhead
Operating Room	237,665	443,116	205,451	8.0
Post Oper. Room	64,378	88,620	24,242	.9
Anesthesiology	167,259	205,017	37,758	1.4
Delivery Room	81,783	155,071	73,288	2.8
Radiology	379,921	500,922	121,001	4.6
Laboratory	504,405	845,294	340,889	13.0
EEG	13,361	20,641	7,280	.3
EKG	75,294	114,446	39,152	1.5
Physical Therapy	29,285	54,694	25,409	.9
Central Supply	81,942	59,660	(22,282)	(.8)
Respiratory Therapy	52,356	74,250	21,894	.8
IV Therapy	122,841	160,851	38,010	1.5
Pharmacy	185,238	175,178	(10,060)	(.4)
Emergency Room	83,659	146,660	63,001	2.4
Isotopes	90,286	106,626	16,340	.6
Mental Health	(6,924)	7,732	14,656	.6
Radiation Therapy	9,591	12,734	3,143	.1
Nonmaternity Nur.	1,095,663	2,514,349	1,418,686	54.4
Maternity	74,660	170,726	96,066	3.8
Newborn	67,032	119,305	52,273	2.0
Outpatient	16,655	56,040	39,385	1.6
Total	3,426,350	6,031,932	2,605,582	100.0

Source: Reprinted from *Understanding Hospital Financial Management*, 2nd ed., by A.G. Herkimer, Jr., p. 182, Aspen Publishers, Inc., © 1986.

Compared with a comprehensive cost finding study, the short-formula 1 method of cost finding requires a minimal amount of time and is still fairly accurate. However, if there has been a major statistical or expense distribution (e.g., increased square footage of a department), the overhead ratio(s) must be adjusted to compensate for the change(s). To assure statistical validity, a comprehensive cost finding should be completed at least once a year.

The type of cost finding method that should be used depends on management's objectives. If a detailed and accurate study which can withstand external review and scrutiny is required, one of the more traditional methods should be chosen. However, if a reasonable approximation will satisfy management's objectives, then an abbreviated cost finding process will suffice. There is no need here to debate the validity of any methodology or describe how to perform a comprehensive cost finding program, for there are many books written on the subject. The purpose of this book is to acquaint the reader with the technique and to encourage the use of some form of cost finding in budgeting and price setting.

Table 9-2 Application of Short-Formula 1 Method of Cost Finding to the Revenue-Producing Departmental Operations for the Three-Month Period Ending December 31, 19x5

Department	% of Gross Charges(A)	Overhead Ratio	Gross Charges to Patients	Less: Deductions & Allowances(B)	Net Charges to Patients	Direct Expense	Indirect Expense(C)	Total Expense	Net Gain or (Loss)
Operating Room	7.4	8.0	$ 509,583	$ 48,444	$ 461,139	$ 261,143	$ 174,385	$ 435,528	$ 25,611
Postoperative Room	1.5	0.9	101,913	9,820	92,093	70,815	19,618	90,433	1,660
Anesthesiology	3.4	1.4	235,770	22,258	213,512	183,985	30,517	214,502	(990)
Delivery Room	1.9	2.8	132,332	12,438	119,894	89,960	61,035	150,995	(31,101)
Radiology	8.4	4.6	576,060	54,990	521,070	417,913	100,271	518,184	2,886
Laboratory	14.2	13.0	972,088	92,960	879,128	554,845	283,375	838,220	40,908
EEG	0.3	.3	23,737	1,964	21,773	14,697	6,539	21,236	537
EKG	1.9	1.5	131,613	12,438	119,175	82,823	32,697	115,520	3,655
Physical Therapy	0.9	.9	62,898	5,892	57,006	32,213	19,618	51,831	5,175
Central Supply	1.0	(.8)	68,909	6,546	62,363	90,136	(17,438)	72,698	(10,335)
Respiratory Therapy	1.2	.8	85,388	7,856	77,532	57,592	17,438	75,030	2,502
IV Therapy	2.7	1.5	184,979	17,675	167,304	135,125	32,697	167,822	(518)
Pharmacy	2.9	(.4)	201,455	18,985	182,470	203,760	(8,719)	195,041	(12,571)
Emergency Room	2.4	2.4	168,659	15,711	152,948	92,025	52,315	144,340	8,608
Isotopes	1.8	.6	122,620	11,784	110,836	99,315	13,079	112,394	(1,558)
Mental Health	0.1	.6	8,892	655	8,237	7,616	13,079	20,695	(12,458)
Radiation Therapy	0.2	.1	14,644	1,309	13,335	10,550	2,180	12,730	605
Nonmaternity Nursing	42.0	54.4	2,891,501	274,952	2,616,549	1,205,229	1,185,817	2,391,046	225,503
Maternity Nursing	2.8	3.8	196,335	18,330	178,005	82,126	82,833	164,959	13,046
Newborn Nursing	2.1	2.0	137,200	13,748	123,453	73,735	43,596	117,331	6,122
Outpatient	0.9	1.6	64,446	5,892	58,554	18,320	34,877	53,197	5,357
Total	100.0	100.0	$6,891,022	$654,647	$6,236,375	$3,783,923	$2,179,809	$5,963,732	$272,643

(A) Source: Percent of departmental charges to total gross charges to patients.
   For example: operating room $\frac{\$ 509,583}{\$6,891,022} = .074$ or 7.4%.

(B) Source: Departmental percent of total gross charges to patients multiplied by total deductions and allowances.
   For example: operating room .074 × $654,647 = $48,444.

(C) Source: Total indirect expense represents the balance of expenses after direct expenses have been deducted.
   For example: $5,963,732 less $3,783,923 = $2,179,809.
   Departmental indirect expenses are computed by multiplying overhead ratio by total indirect expenses.
   For example: operating room .08 × $2,179,809 = $174,385.

Source: Reprinted from *Understanding Hospital Financial Management*, 2nd ed., by A.G. Herkimer, Jr., p. 187, Aspen Publishers, Inc., © 1986.

DEPARTMENTAL CONTRIBUTION

In addition to evaluating the profitability of a revenue-producing department, a department can be assessed by determining how much revenue, either gross or net, it contributes to the institution's overhead expenses. Gross revenue is based on the department's published charges or prices before any provision has been made for contractual, charity, and administrative allowances and bad debts. The net contribution is computed after these provisions have been deducted from the gross revenue. In both cases, the contribution is the department's revenue surplus after subtracting its direct expenses. For example, if the gross patient revenue of Hometown Memorial Hospital's laboratory department was $8,345,987 and its related direct operating expenses totaled $6,532,178, the department's gross contribution to the hospital's total overhead would be calculated as follows:

Description	Amount	Percent
Gross patient revenue	$8,345,987	100.00%
Less direct operating expenses	6,532,178	78.27
Gross contribution	$1,813,809	21.73%

Departmental contributions do not have to be uniform throughout the institution. The rate of contribution depends on management's philosophy. For example, in the expectation of increasing inpatient day volume, management may decide to operate the medical and surgical routine nursing department at a very low contribution level so that the room and board rate is low enough to attract the comparative shopper. On the other hand, since it is relatively difficult to compare operating room fees among health care facilities, management may decide to expect a higher contribution from its surgical suite. It is important only that the combined contribution of the revenue-producing departments be sufficient to cover the institution's overhead expenses and to generate management's desired net operating profit (see Table 9-3).

BREAK-EVEN ANALYSIS

The evaluation techniques described to this point are used to assess the efficiency of a revenue-producing department. Break-even analysis is a procedure which evaluates the price of a department's production unit and determines its break-even point as well. The break-even concept requires that all departmental expenses be classified as either fixed or variable. Comparatively speaking, the higher the amount of the fixed expenses, the greater the sales volume required to break even (see Figure 9-1). Conversely, the lower the amount of fixed expenses, the lower the level of patient services required to break even (see Figure 9-2).

Table 9-3 Comparative Analysis of Contributions of the Medical and Surgical Nursing, Operating Rooms, and Pharmacy Departments as of June 30, 19x5

| | | (in thousands) | | |
Department	Total	M & S Nursing	Operating Rooms	Pharmacy
Net revenue	$20,753	$10,543	$3,632	$6,578
Direct expenses	13,724	8,965	1,462	3,297
Contribution to overhead	$ 7,029	$ 1,578	$2,170	$3,281
Contribution margin to overhead	33.87%	14.97%	59.75%	49.88%

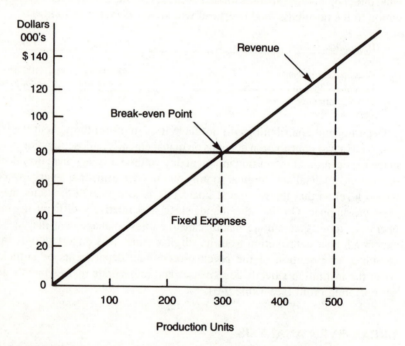

Figure 9-1 High Fixed Expense Break-even Point (Excluding Variable Expenses)

Source: Adapted from *Understanding Hospital Financial Management*, 2nd ed., by A.G. Herkimer, Jr., p. 55, Aspen Publishers, Inc., © 1986.

In evaluating a department, its contribution to the institution's overhead is the financial or percentage difference between the department's total revenue and its total operating expenses. In determining a department's break-even sales or volume, the contribution is the dollar difference between the total net charge or

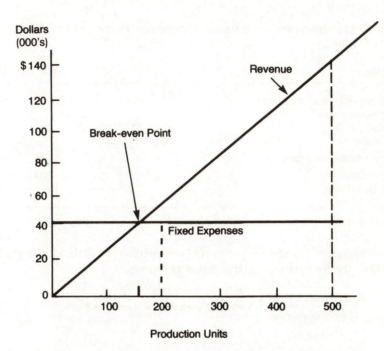

Figure 9-2 Low Fixed Expense Break-even Point (Excluding Variable Expenses)

Source: Adapted from *Understanding Hospital Financial Management*, 2nd ed., by A.G. Herkimer, Jr., p. 55, Aspen Publishers, Inc., © 1986.

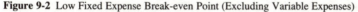

price and the related variable expenses for one production unit. The contribution margin is the percentage expression of this amount (see Table 9-4). A departmental production unit's contribution and contribution margin are used to determine a department's break-even point.

Using the data in Table 9-4 (with $50,000 as fixed departmental expenses), the following two formulas can be used to compute the department's break-even point:

1. Break-even volume:

$$\frac{\text{Fixed expenses}}{\text{Contribution per unit}} = \text{break-even volume of production units}$$

or

$$\frac{\$50,000}{\$4} = 12,500 \text{ production units}$$

Table 9-4 Contribution Analysis of Radiology Department Production Unit as of June 30, 19x8

Description		Total	Percent
Net charge per relative value unit		$25.00	100%
Variable expenses			
Labor	$17.50		
Nonlabor	3.50		
Total variable expenses		21.00	84
Contribution		$ 4.00	NA
Contribution margin		NA	16%

If management desires a departmental contribution to overhead or a profit of $150,000, the formula would be adjusted as follows:

$$\frac{\text{Fixed expenses} + \text{profit}}{\text{Contribution per unit}} = \text{break-even volume of production units}$$

or

$$\frac{\$50,000 + \$150,000}{\$4} = 50{,}000 \text{ production units with profit provision}$$

2. Break-even sales:

$$\frac{\text{Fixed expenses}}{\text{Contribution margin}} = \text{break-even sales}$$

or

$$\frac{\$50,000}{.16} = \$312{,}500$$

If, as in the above example, management expects an additional $150,000 from the department, the formula would be adjusted as follows:

$$\frac{\text{Fixed expenses} + \text{profit}}{\text{Contribution margin}} = \text{break-even sales with profit provision}$$

or

$$\frac{\$50,000 + \$150,000}{.16} = \$1{,}250{,}000$$

The data used in the above computations are laid out below. (The data in the "Break-even Volume" column are displayed in the graph in Figure 9-3.)

Description	Amount per Unit	Percent	Break-even Volume	Total Volume and Profit
Volume	1		12,500	50,000
Price/sales	$25.00	100%	$312,500	$1,250,000
Variable expenses	21.00	84	262,500	1,050,000
Contribution	$ 4.00	16%	$ 50,000	$ 200,000
Fixed expenses			50,000	50,000
Profit			$ 0	$ 150,000

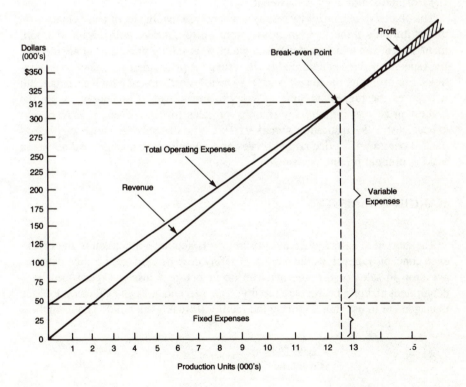

Figure 9-3 Graphic Break-even Analysis of Radiology Department for Period Ending June 30, 19x3

The most useful purpose of break-even analysis is as a decision-making aid in pricing health care services.[5] Since it is almost mandatory that health care institutions select profitable product lines, it is important that their determined prices recover their operating expenses and make any desired profits.

SENSITIVITY TESTING

Sensitivity testing, an extended variation of break-even analysis, is the process of taking known factors and evaluating them under changing conditions. All but one of the factors in the break-even formula are fixed by either budgetary restrictions or management decisions. The one remaining element in the formula is *price*. Since price is the only variable factor, it lends itself uniquely to sensitivity testing. Table 9-5 is an example of price sensitivity testing for Hometown Memorial Hospital's radiology department.

The objective of sensitivity testing is to analyze the impact of price changes on the institution's or the department's operating profit. Armed with this information, management can then best determine which final selling price is most appropriate for a specific service or commodity. In setting the price, there are many considerations. For example, the lowest price may be the most attractive for the market, but it requires the highest volume of sales to break even. Conversely, while the highest price may require fewer units of sales to break even, it may be too expensive for the institution's market. This type of analysis, which can be expanded over a wide price range, serves as a guide to management and assists in making optimal pricing decisions.

MARGIN OF SAFETY

The margin of safety evaluation technique is another application of the break-even concept. It develops the margin of safety drop percentage, i.e., the percentage drop in sales or revenue that can occur before a loss is experienced by a department and/or a health care facility. This percentage is an evaluation tool for management to use in monitoring the facility's break-even point. The formula is

$$\frac{\text{Desired profit}}{\text{Contribution}} = \text{margin of safety (MS)}$$

Using the data in Table 9-5 for price option 1, the margin of safety is computed as follows:

Table 9-5 Price Sensitivity Testing for the Radiology Department as of June 30, 19x3

| | Price Option | | | | |
Description	(1)	(2)	(3)	(4)	(5)
Unit price	$ 25.00	$ 23.00	$ 27.00	$ 29.00	$ 31.00
Variable expenses	21.00	21.00	21.00	21.00	21.00
Contribution	$ 4.00	$ 2.00	$ 6.00	$ 8.00	$ 10.00
Contribution margin	16.0%	8.7%	22.2%	27.6%	32.3%
Fixed expenses	$ 50,000	$ 50,000	$ 50,000	$ 50,000	$ 50,000
Desired profit	$ 150,000	$ 150,000	$150,000	$150,000	$150,000
Break-even Only					
B-E volume units	12,500	25,000	8,333	6,250	5,000
B-E sales	$ 312,500	$ 575,000	$224,991	$181,250	$155,000
Proof:					
B-E sales	$ 312,500	$ 575,000	$224,991	$181,250	$155,000
Variable expenses	262,500	525,000	174,993	131,250	105,000
Contribution to fixed expenses	$ 50,000	$ 50,000	$ 49,998	$ 50,000	$ 50,000
Break-even with Profit					
B-E profit volume	50,000	100,000	33,333	25,000	20,000
B-E profit sales	$1,250,000	$2,300,000	$899,991	$725,000	$620,000
Proof:					
B-E profit sales	$1,250,000	$2,300,000	$899,991	$725,000	$620,000
Variable expenses	1,050,000	2,100,000	699,993	525,000	420,000
Contribution to fixed expenses and profit	$ 200,000	$ 200,000	$199,998	$200,000	$200,000

Break-even volume with profit	50,000
Break-even sales with profit	$1,250,000
Variable expenses	$1,050,000
Desired profit	$ 150,000
Contribution	$ 200,000
Contribution margin	16%

Using the margin of safety formula,

$$\frac{\$150,000}{\$200,000} = MS$$

or

$$75\% = MS$$

The margin of safety is verified as follows:

Description	Desired Results	Percent	75% Decreased Volume
Volume	50,000	NA	37,500
Unit price	$25.00	NA	$25.00
Unit variable expense	$21.00	NA	$21.00
B-E sales	$1,250,000	100%	$937,500
Variable expenses	$1,050,000	84%	$787,500
Contribution	$ 200,000	16%	$ 50,000
Fixed expenses	$ 50,000	NA	$ 50,000
Profit	$ 150,000	NA	$ 0

The break-even point for this facility is that point where the revenue and the total fixed and variable expenses are the same, i.e., at a volume of 37,500 production units. Any decrease in sales volume results in an operating loss while an increase results in profits.

EVALUATING CAPITAL INVESTMENTS

The evaluation techniques which we have discussed thus far relate only to a health care institution's operations. In this section, methods to evaluate capital expenditures are presented.

Conceptually, the net present value (NPV) or discounted cash flow analysis surpasses most other capital evaluation techniques, but even this method must be supported by a reasonable degree of common sense.[6] Most capital evaluation systems analyze capital investments

1. to determine whether the original capital investment and its related operating expenses are recovered within the useful life of the investment
2. to determine the length of time required to recover the original investment and its related operating expenses

Ultimately, management wants to know what rate of return it can expect to realize in addition to recovering the initial cost of the investment and its related operating expenses.

Before examining the NPV methodology, we will examine the more traditional methods of *payback* and *bailout*.

For the purpose of illustrating the basic payback approach, assume that the original investment (I) of $250,000 is projected so that it annually generates a net opportunity or profit (O) of $50,000. The payback formula is

$$\frac{\text{Investment (I)}}{\text{Opportunity (O)}} = \text{Payback (P)}$$

The payback period (P) is calculated as follows:

$$\frac{\$250,000}{\$\ 50,000} = 5 \text{ (years)}$$

The bailout approach considers the salvage value of the capital investment. Using the same investment information as above, assume that the salvage value is $150,000 at the end of the first year and that this amount declines at the rate of $25,000 per year thereafter. The bailout payback schedule is computed as follows:

At End of Year	Cumulative Opportunities	+	Salvage Value	=	Cumulative Payback
1	$ 50,000	+	$150,000	=	$200,000
2	100,000	+	125,000	=	225,000
3	150,000	+	100,000	=	250,000
4	200,000	+	75,000	=	275,000
5	250,000	+	50,000	=	300,000
6	300,000	+	25,000	=	325,000
7	350,000	+	0	=	350,000

The cumulative payback total at the end of the third year is $250,000, which is equal to the original investment. Therefore, using the bailout payback methodology, management could theoretically scrap the investment and recover the original cost and the related operating expenses.

Unlike the payback systems, the NPV method of evaluating capital investments assumes that the use of money has cost. Cash received today has more value than a year from now, especially in an inflationary economy. NPV weighs the time value of money at an interest rate of return selected by management.[7] Basically, there are three types of NPV opportunities or decisions:

1. A positive NPV investment increases the value of the organization even after the original investment has been recovered at the rate of return and over the payback period desired by management.
2. A negative NPV investment decreases the value of the organization before recovery of the original investment at the rate of return and over the payback period desired by management.
3. A zero NPV investment produces only enough operational cash flow to match exactly the organization's capital overall. These types of investment result in a significant positive amount of accounting income or profit.[8]

Exhibit 9-4 is an NPV analysis of the capital investment considered above in the discussion of the payback methods for evaluating investments. According to the analysis, the organization will experience a $49,400 negative NPV, a 6 percent rate of return (as developed below), and still realize a negative NPV of $39,400.

Since management considers the useful life of this investment to be only five years, it appears to be a "no buy" decision.

Year	Cash Flow	NPV @ 6%	NPV Value
19x1	$ 50,000	.943	$ 47,150
19x2	50,000	.890	44,500
19x3	50,000	.840	42,000
19x4	50,000	.792	39,600
19x5	50,000	.747	37,350
Total	$250,000		$210,600
Original investment			250,000
Negative NPV			$ 39,400

Exhibit 9-4 Net Present Value Capital Investment Analysis

Hometown Memorial Hospital
Hometown, U.S.A.

Net Present Value Analysis of Capital Investment
as of June 30, 19x5

Original Investment: $250,000
Useful Life: 5 years
Annual Opportunity: $50,000
Desired Rate of Return: 9%

| Year | Discounted Value @ 8% | Net Present Value | Year End Cash Flows | | | | |
			19x1	19x2	19x3	19x4	19x5
19x1	.926	$ 46,300	$50,000				
19x2	.875	43,750		$50,000			
19x3	.794	39,700			$50,000		
19x4	.735	36,750				$50,000	
19x5	.681	34,050					$50,000
NPV cash flow		$200,600					
Original investment		250,000					
Negative NPV		$ 49,400					

A capital investment should never be evaluated using only one method. The techniques discussed in this chapter provide the decision maker(s) with points of reference that will be helpful in reaching a decision, but none of these methods contains the most important elements: common sense, human intuition, and the consideration of each capital investment on the basis of its own merits and its worth to the organization.

BUDGET BALANCERS AND THE FINAL BUDGET

Budget balancers are strategies which management devises after evaluating the ability of each revenue-producing department to generate the desired operating profit. Exhibit 9-5 lists Hometown Memorial Hospital's budget balancers for the

---

Exhibit 9-5 Proposed Budget Balancers

Hometown Memorial Hospital
Hometown, U.S.A.

Reconciliation of Preliminary Budget's Operating Loss
with Proposed Budget Balancers
for the Budget Year Ending December 31, 19x6

Preliminary Budget Operating Loss	$1,750,000
Budget Balancers:	
1. Increase medical & surgical room rates by $10 per patient day.	
56,476 patient days × $10.	$564,760
2. Increase operating room rate by $ .50 per Operating Room minute.	
384,792 OR minutes @ $ .50	192,396
3. Increase emergency service routine admission by $20.	
23,465 admissions @ $20	469,300
4. Increase laboratory relative value unit (RVU) rates by $ .10 each.	
3,178,945 RVUs @ $ .10	317,894
5. Increase radiology RVU rate by $ .15.	
1,765,987 RVUs @ $ .15	264,898
6. Increase ICU/CCU room rate $25 per patient day.	
28,654 patient days @ $25	716,350
Total budget balancers	2,525,598
Total budgeted operating profit	$ 950,598
Desired operating profit	$ 900,000
Contingency	$ 50,598

budget year ending December 31, 19x6. When the budget balancers have been approved by the governing board, they should be incorporated into the preliminary budget; then the final (master) budget is generated.

NOTES

1. Allen G. Herkimer, Jr., *Understanding Hospital Financial Management*, 2d ed. (Rockville, Md.: Aspen, 1986), 173–174.

2. Ibid.

3. Ibid., 176–80.

4. Ibid., 181–82, 187.

5. William O. Cleverly, *Handbook of Health Care Accounting and Finance* (Rockville, Md.: Aspen, 1982), 175.

6. Herkimer, *Understanding Hospital Financial Management*, 290.

7. Ibid., 290–300.

8. Hugh W. Long, "The Future of Financing Decisions in the Health Care Industry," in *Health Care Financial Management in the 1980's*, ed. J.B. Silvers, William N. Zelman, Charles N. Kahn III (Ann Arbor, Mich.: AUPHA Press, 1983), 32–33.

Cash Flow Forecast

10

The cash flow forecast is usually the last document to be prepared during the budget development process, and yet it is one of the primary reasons the budget is constructed. It forecasts to management what the cash position of the organization is well in advance of any dramatic cash shortfall or whether there will be an excess of idle cash available for investment. Knowing an institution's cash position well in advance helps to reassure management that the organization will stay financially viable and be able to pay its employees, replenish its inventories, repay its financial obligations, and have sufficient additional cash to allow it to expand and to grow. Inadequate cash planning is often a major cause of business failure.[1]

A well-prepared cash flow forecast tells management when and for how long the organization is going to experience the need for additional cash or the need to invest excess cash.[2] Knowing about these conditions will assist management in optimizing the organization's cash resources. For example, if management knows well in advance when the organization is going to require additional cash funds, it can review alternative sources of cash, decide which is best, and do whatever is necessary to obtain that cash. On the other hand, if management knows when to expect excess cash, it can investigate and evaluate a variety of capital investment options and select the one which optimizes the extra funds.

At this point, it is important to compare the operating revenue and expense budgets with the cash flow forecast. The operating budgets are based on the accrual accounting concepts and do not include any accounting for capital expenditures. The only capital-related expense in the operating budgets is the noncash provision for depreciation. The operating budgets project only the organization's operating profits or losses and do not reveal management's cash requirements or cash position. The cash flow forecast, on the other hand, projects only the institution's cash inflows and outflows, including capital investments and borrowings, and is not concerned with operating profits or losses.

159

FIVE-POINT CASH FLOW FORECAST MODEL

The cash flow report design must be one which best fits management's needs. Most cash flow models forecast an institution's monthly cash flow using five basic components (see also Table 10-1):

1. beginning balance
2. cash inflows
3. cash-on-hand
4. cash outflows
5. ending balance

Cash flow forecasts are usually generated for the institution as a whole, but a departmental cash flow analysis can be developed if a department manager wants to project the department's cash impact on, contribution to, or drainage from the institution. If this is desired, institutional averages such as provision for allowances from gross patient revenues, cash collection on net patient revenues, and payments on vendor trade payables may be used to arrive at a reasonable cash impact.

BEGINNING BALANCE

The beginning balance represents the amount in the institution's bank account at the start of the cash flow forecast. This amount may be identified either from the organization's reconciled bank statement or from the organization's related general ledger account. Obviously, if the beginning balance is incorrect, the accuracy of the forecast is questionable.

CASH INFLOWS

Patient accounts receivable are generally a health care organization's largest source of cash inflow.[3] The amount of monthly net patient charges—after provisions for contractual allowance, administrative discounts, and bad debts have been removed—usually serve as the basis for projecting cash flow from patient accounts receivable. This process is discussed later in the chapter.

Borrowing or other outside financing (e.g., loans, mortgages, bonds, stock issues, etc.) constitutes the health care organization's second largest source of cash inflow.[4] Short-term loans are frequently used in the cash flow statement to recognize the need for additional funds.

Table 10-1 Master Cash Flow Forecast for the Budget Year Ending December 31, 19x6

Description	January	February	March	April	May	June	July	August	September	October	November	December	Total
1. Beginning cash balance	$ 10	$ 4	$ 17	$ 17	$ 5	$ 15	$ −6	$ −6	$ 17	$ 11	$ 15	$ 11	$ 10
2. Cash inflows:													
A. Patient receivables	$785	$917	$ 946	$939	$902	$ 833	$799	$815	$815	$ 822	$828	$822	$10223
B. Negotiated contracts (HMOs)	43	44	43	46	45	46	44	46	44	46	46	47	540
C. Other operating sources	39	32	29	25	25	20	21	21	20	26	20	21	299
D. Investment income	5	5	5	5	5	5	5	5	5	5	5	5	60
E. Borrowings (investments and/or paybacks)	15	−115	15	−150	−150	400		75	50	250	−50	−30	310
F. Total cash inflows	$887	$883	$1038	$865	$827	$1304	$869	$962	$934	$1149	$849	$865	$11432
3. Total cash-on-hand	$897	$887	$1055	$882	$832	$1319	$863	$956	$951	$1160	$864	$876	$11442
4. Cash outflows:													
A. Salaries, wages and education-related expenses	$370	$385	$ 400	$407	$407	$ 415	$415	$427	$427	$ 435	$435	$442	$ 4965
B. Programmed expenses	245	205	205	245	205	205	245	205	205	250	205	205	2625
C. Variable operating expenses	153	130	133	175	155	155	159	157	158	160	163	164	1862
D. Funded depreciation	50	50	50	50	50	50	50	50	50	50	50	50	600
E. Capital expenditures	75	100	250	0	0	500	0	100	100	250	0	0	1375
F. Other investments													0
G. Total cash outflows	$893	$870	$1038	$877	$817	$1325	$869	$939	$940	$1145	$853	$861	$11427
5. Ending cash balance	$ 4	$ 17	$ 17	$ 5	$ 15	$ −6	$ −6	$ 17	$ 11	$ 15	$ 11	$ 15	$ 15

An alternate method to listing borrowings as a single line on the forecast statement is to include investments and/or paybacks as well as borrowings on the same line. For example, if the initial calculation of cash-on-hand minus cash outflows shows the resulting ending balance to be negative, this condition would require additional cash (borrowings). On the other hand, if the resulting ending balance is positive, it might be appropriate to invest or pay back some of the excess cash and record this amount on the same line (borrowings/investments) as a negative amount. By using the borrowings/investments as a common line in the cash forecast statement, the user can easily calculate the net amount of borrowings over paybacks or investments. The borrowings/investments line item can also be used as a balancing line item after the ending balance is adjusted to the desired cash position. If, for example, an excess amount of cash appears in the ending balance, invest or pay back a portion on the borrowings/investments line. If there is a cash "shortfall," record the needed cash as a borrowing on the same line, thus maintaining the desired ending bank balance.

The remaining cash inflows to the health care facility are generated from such sources as

- investment income
- gifts and donations
- rentals
- vending machines
- cafeteria sales
- medical record transcriptions
- transfers from the parent corporation

The number of individually identified line items in the cash flow section of the forecast depends on management's "need to know." It is recommended, however, that all items which contribute 5 percent or more to the institution's cash inflow should be included as separate line items on the statement.

CASH-ON-HAND

The cash-on-hand portion of the forecast statement is the total of the month's beginning cash balance and the month's total cash inflows. After the initial calculation, this amount is frequently adjusted on the borrowings/investments line in order to generate the desired ending bank balance for that month.

CASH OUTFLOWS

Cash outflows are generally separated into four major classifications:

1. salaries, wages, and related expenses
2. fixed or programmed expenses
3. variable operation expenses
4. capital expenditures

The cash flow statement in Table 10-1 lists funded depreciation and other investments as well.

A health care institution's largest cash outflows are the monies paid for salaries, wages, and other related expenses, e.g., social security taxes, retirement benefits, health insurance, etc. Although these expenses are usually budgeted on a monthly basis, for cash management purposes they must be planned according to the frequency and to the time of actual cash disbursement to employees, whether it be weekly, biweekly, or monthly.[5]

Both groups of the fixed or programmed expenses and the variable operating expenses are generated from the organization's vendors' accounts payable files; the similarity between these two types of expense is that both are nonsalary related. Programmed expenses, usually a fixed amount regardless of volume of activity, are those for which payment is scheduled at specific times throughout the year, e.g., insurance premiums, mortgage payments, rentals, and leases. Even though the expense for utilities (e.g., electricity, gas, and water) varies rather than being fixed, it is a type of programmed expense which routinely reoccurs and the amounts are fairly predictable. Such types of programmed expense have a top priority for timely payment. (The prioritizing of accounts payable will be discussed later.)

Variable operating expenses, such as food, medical and surgical supplies, pharmaceuticals, etc., tend to vary in direct proportion to an institution's volume of activity. Unlike the salary and programmed expenses, which need routine and prompt payment, the variable operating expenses can be scheduled for payment over a period of time.

Capital expenditures represent most of the manageable cash outflow items in terms of time available to disburse cash, and they can usually be delayed without jeopardizing operations. Consequently, management can place a "hold" on purchasing any capital asset until the institution's cash position is more favorable. Conversely, if there is an excess of operating cash, appropriate capital expenditures (investments) probably should be made.[6]

The cash outflows include all of a health care institution's operating expenses, together with its capital expenditures, except its provision for depreciation. This is excluded because the provision for depreciation is an accounting procedure which amortizes a capital investment over a period of time and does not require a cash outlay. If, however, it is management's policy to fund (invest) some or all of the provision for depreciation for replacement of capital assets, this amount should be distributed as a single line item as "funded depreciation" (see Table 10-1, line 4D). The cash flow accounting for the acquisition of a capital investment is recorded in the cash flow statement only when cash is planned for disbursement.

ENDING BALANCE

The monthly ending balance is computed by subtracting the month's cash outflows from the amount of its cash-on-hand; this becomes the subsequent month's beginning balance. The budget year's total cash inflows and outflows are summarized in the extreme right-hand "total" column (see Table 10-1). The beginning balance in the total column must be identical to the starting balance in the first month's column. Likewise, the ending balance of the last month is identical to the total column's ending balance. The ideal ending balance of the operating cash account is zero. This would mean that the institution's management is optimizing the operating cash by either paying for the day-to-day operations and/or investing the balance in some kind of capital investment, e.g., capital asset, money market fund, etc. Obviously, maintaining a zero or near-zero balance may not always be possible. The monthly ending balance, however, should be maintained at a minimal amount in order to obtain maximum use of the funds. For illustrative purposes only, the monthly ending balances in the master cash flow statement (see Table 10-1) were deliberately programmed to range from negative $6,000 to a positive balance of $17,000.

FORECASTING PATIENT ACCOUNTS RECEIVABLE

The next step in cash forecasting after the beginning bank balance has been identified is to analyze cash inflows from patient accounts receivable. This process is based on the institution's monthly net revenues or patient charges. As stated earlier, net patient revenues represent the residue after all provisions for contractual allowances, administrative and charity discounts, and bad debts have been deducted from gross patient revenues or charges. Net revenues represent the maximum amount of cash the health care organization can expect to receive from its patient services.

Most health care institutions do not expect to be paid in full at the time of the patient's discharge. Occasionally, the patient is a "self-pay" patient who is prepared to pay in full, but the vast majority of patients have some kind of health care insurance. Insurance companies or third party payers have many types of payment systems (e.g., per diem, per case, per charges, percent of charges, etc.) as well as a variety of payment patterns.

The provisions for allowances and deductions from gross patient revenues usually compensate for the variations in payment systems, but the payment patterns of the third party payers can, and do, vary greatly. For example, one paying agent may pay its portion within 30 days whereas another may take 60 days or more. It is therefore imperative that the payment patterns of each paying agent, including each self-pay patient, be analyzed so as to determine time-lag factors.

A patient accounts receivable time-lag factor is the historical payment pattern a paying agent (or agents) used to liquidate a patient account receivable. In some cases, an account may be totally paid by one agent, but most accounts are the joint responsibility of the patient, the insured (subscriber) and/or the insured's family, and a third party guarantor. The payment pattern of such an account might be analyzed as shown in Table 10-2.

The process of analyzing each paying agent's payment pattern is extremely time consuming. In addition, these patterns can vary according to external economic factors such as inflation, local economics, interest rates, budget deficits, etc. For this reason, the best approach is to conduct periodic statistical samplings of the institution's total patient accounts receivable (e.g., once every six months). The results of such a sampling might resemble the percent analysis of payment patterns illustrated in Table 10-3.

After the payment patterns have been identified for each paying agent, the next step is to determine the net revenue from each agent. Since every paying agent has unique payment methods, each will require a specific provision for contractual allowances, administrative and charity discounts, and bad debts to be deducted from its gross patient revenues (see Table 10-4). Note that ABC/HMO's payment method, per capita, has no relevance to the amount of services rendered to its members. Therefore, this paying agent's cash inflows to the institution should be recorded as a separate line item (see Table 10-1, line 2C).

Table 10-2 Analysis of the Payment Patterns of the Net Patient Accounts Receivable Discharged on September 30, 19x5

Guarantor	Time of Payment	Payment Amount	Percent
Patient	Prepayment at admission	$ 500	5.0%
Insurance	30 days after discharge	7,500	75.0
Patient	60 days after discharge	1,000	10.0
Patient	90 days after discharge	750	7.5
Patient	120 days after discharge	250	2.5
Total net patient revenue		$10,000	100.0

Table 10-3 Percent Analysis of Payment Patterns by Paying Agents from 200 Randomly
Selected Patient Accounts Receivable as of September 30, 19x5

Paying Agent	% of Payments Received in Days after Discharge						
	0–30	31–60	61–90	91–120	121–150	over 150	Total
Medicare	55	25	15	5	—	—	100.0
Medicaid	10	15	25	30	15	5	100.0
Blue Cross	30	35	20	10	5	—	100.0
ABC/HMO	not applicable: receive $50 per month per member						
Commercial insurance	20	30	25	20	5	—	100.0
Self-pay & others	15	25	25	15	10	10	100.0

Table 10-4 Percent Analysis of Patient Charges for the Six-Month Period Ending
September 30, 19x5

Paying Agent	Gross Revenue	Less Deductibles	Net Revenue
Medicare	100.0%	15.0%	85.0%
Medicaid	100.0	35.0	65.0
Blue Cross	100.0	12.0	88.0
ABC/HMO	100.0	10.0	90.0
Commercial insurance	100.0	5.0	95.0
Self-pay & others	100.0	15.0	85.0

Table 10-5 is an extended analysis of patient gross revenues by paying agent as
they relate to the institution's total gross patient revenues.

There are at least two methods to forecast cash inflows from net patient
revenues. The first method is to calculate anticipated gross revenues by individual
paying agent, deduct the unique provision for deductibles (see Table 10-4), and
project the cash inflows based on the statistical sampling of the payment patterns
(see Table 10-3). Assuming that Hometown Memorial Hospital's projected

Table 10-5 Percent Analysis of Gross Patient Revenues by Paying Agent as of
September 30, 19x5

Paying Agent	% of Gross Revenue
Medicare	35%
Medicaid	10
Blue Cross	30
ABC/HMO	5
Commercial insurance	15
Self-pay & others	5
Total	100

annual total gross patient revenue is $12,000,000 and using the distribution in Table 10-5, each paying agent's annual share of the net patient revenue is computed as shown in Table 10-6. Using the individual cash forecasting method, each of these annual revenues requires monthly distribution for the budget year. This type of cash flow projection is not examined in this text. Instead, we shall use the weighted average method for all payers.

Although the individual paying agent approach may be preferable, another cash forecasting method uses an institution's weighted average for its provision for deductibles when computing net patient revenues. After the deductible percentage has been determined, a weighted average of monthly collection percentage of the net patient revenue is calculated as follows. Let MC be the weighted monthly collection percent, let R be the paying agent's share of net revenues, let $(R \times MC^1)$ be the weighted percentage (first month), and let $\Sigma(R \times MC^1)$ be the sum total of the first month's weighted percentages. An illustration of the application of the formula and the computation of the first month's weighted collection pattern percentage is shown below:

Paying Agent	Percent of Net Revenue (R)	×	Percent Collected (MC¹)	=	Weighted Percent
Medicare	.348	×	.55	=	.191
Medicaid	.077	×	.10	=	.008
Blue Cross	.309	×	.30	=	.093
ABC/HMO	NA		NA		NA
Commercial insurance	.166	×	.20	=	.033
Self-pay & others	.050	×	.15	=	.008
Total					.333

Table 10-6 Cash Flow Forecast from Net Patient Revenue by Paying Agent for the Budget Year Ending December 31, 19x6

	Gross Revenue		Deductions		Net Revenue		% of Net Rev.
Paying Agent	%	$	%	$	%	$	
Medicare	35%	$ 4,200	15%	$ 630	85%	$ 3,570	34.8%
Medicaid	10	1,200	35	420	65	780	7.7
Blue Cross	30	3,600	12	430	88	3,170	30.9
ABC/HMO	5	600	10	60	90	540	5.0
Commercial insurance	15	1,800	5	90	95	1,710	16.6
Self-pay & others	5	600	15	90	85	510	5.0
Total	100%	$12,000	14.3%	$1,720	85.7%	$10,280	100.0%
Less ABC/HMO						540*	
Adjusted Total						$ 9,740*	

(in thousands of dollars)

*The collection of these receivables is distributed by the month in Table 10-9.

The weighted amount of 33.3 percent (.333) is the percentage of monthly net patient charges which can reasonably be expected to be collected during the first month (0–30 days after discharge), based on the most recent patient accounts payment pattern analysis. The worksheet in Table 10-7 is the computation table of the monthly weighted average of collection or payment patterns of the hospital's net patient revenues or charges. A summary of the monthly weighted average of payment patterns is shown in Table 10-8.

To apply this schedule of weighted average payment patterns, assume that the annual gross patient revenue is 12 million dollars, as identified in Table 10-6. Further assume that one-twelfth of the net patient revenues of $10,280,000 ($856,666) is the hospital's net revenue for the first month of the budget year. Using these assumptions, the cash inflow from this month's net revenue would be collected over the subsequent months in the following collection (payment) pattern:

Month	Range of Days after Discharge	Weighted Average	Monthly Cash Collections
1	0–30	33.3%	$285,270
2	31–60	26.9	230,443
3	61–90	18.7	160,197
4	91–120	11.2	95,946
5	121–150	4.0	34,267
6	151 & over	0.9	7,710
Subtotal			$813,833
Due from ABC/HMO			42,833
Total			$856,666

Continuing the example, Table 10-9 is a spreadsheet of the monthly payment patterns and total collections from net patient revenues which are to be transferred to the master cash flow forecast in Table 10-1, line 2A. Since the example concerns the beginning of the hospital's cash flow forecasting process, the spreadsheet lists $1,500,000 as the hospital's current net patient accounts receivable.

OTHER CASH FLOWS

Other cash inflows might include gifts, donations, rentals, vending machines, sales of medical transcriptions, sale of scrap, and other items too numerous to list. For the purpose of this study, the figures listed in line 2C of Table 10-1 should be taken to reflect the total other operating income of Hometown Memorial Hospital for the budget year ending December 31, 19x6, as displayed in Table 10-10. It should be further assumed that the hospital expects to generate an average of $5,000 per month from its current investment portfolio (see Table 10-1, line 2D).

Table 10-7 Worksheet for the Computation of Hometown Memorial Hospital's Weighted Average Collection Percentage or Payment Patterns of Net Patient Revenue as of September 30, 19x5

(Each period cell shows the monthly payment pattern percentage / the weighted collection value.)

Paying Agent	% Net Rev.*	Number Days after Discharge/Months†					
		0–30 (1)	31–60 (2)	61–90 (3)	91–120 (4)	121–150 (5)	151 & over (6)
Medicare	34.8%	55% / 19.1%	25% / 8.7%	15% / 5.2%	5% / 1.7%	— / —	— / —
Medicaid	7.7	10 / 0.8	15 / 1.2	25 / 1.9	30 / 2.3	15% / 1.2%	5% / 0.4%
Blue Cross	30.9	30 / 9.3	35 / 10.8	20 / 6.2	10 / 3.1	5 / 1.5	— / —
Com. insur.	16.6	20 / 3.3	30 / 5.0	25 / 4.2	20 / 3.3	5 / 0.8	— / —
Self-pay	5.0	15 / 0.8	25 / 1.2	25 / 1.2	15 / 0.8	10 / 0.5	10 / 0.5
Subtotal	95.0	33.3	26.9	18.7	11.2	4.0	0.9
ABC/HMO	5.0	to be distributed on separate line as monthly premiums are expected to be collected					
Total	100.0	33.3	26.9	18.7	11.2	4.0	0.9

*The source for percentage of net revenues before 5 percent deduction for anticipated amount from ABC/HMO is Table 10-6, column 8.
†The source for monthly percentages of payment received (R) per paying agent is Table 10-3.

Table 10-8 Monthly Weighted Average Payment Pattern of Net Patient Revenues as of
September 30, 19x5

Month	Range of Days after Discharge	Weighted Average Payment Pattern
1	0–30	33.3%
2	31–60	26.9
3	61–90	18.7
4	91–120	11.2
5	121–150	4.0
6	151 & over	0.9

As previously discussed, the cash inflow item entitled borrowings (see Table 10-1, line 2E) serves as the balancing account in order to maintain the desired ending cash balance.

Even though most health care institutions use the accural accounting system, the analysis of cash outflows must be forecast based strictly on the cash that is actually distributed out of the institution. This is especially important where salaries, wages, and other related expenses are concerned.

Many health care institutions maintain a special imprest cash account for the disbursement of payroll checks. This imprest fund maintains a fixed amount (e.g., $10,000) and is routinely reimbursed from the organization's operating cash account in the exact amount(s) to be disbursed, thus maintaining the original fixed sum. In addition, separate checks may be drawn from the operating fund and deposited in the payroll account to cover taxes and other related expenses. For the purpose of this study, the salary and wage analysis in Table 10-11 includes all salaries and related expenses which are recorded in Table 10-1, line 4A. This table shows that Hometown Memorial Hospital pays its employees on the 1st and the 15th day of every month, thus facilitating the cash forecasting, because the accrued payroll expenses are actually disbursed during the month of record.

Programmed or fixed expenses do not vary substantially regardless of the volume of an organization's activity. These expenses might include items such as mortgage payments, utility bills, insurance, rents, and leases. A summary of these expenses is presented in Table 10-12 and the totals are recorded in line 4B of Table 10-1.

Capital expenditures are generated from the capital expenditure plan, as discussed in Chapter 5. For the purpose of the cash flow forecast, they are summarized in Table 10-13, and recorded in line 4E of Table 10-1.

A full portion or more of the sum allocated to the institution's provision for depreciation should be routinely invested to assure that funds are available for the purchase of capital assets. In this study, a monthly amount of $50,000 is programmed in Table 10-1, line 4D.

Table 10-9 Spreadsheet of Monthly Payments from Net Patient Accounts Receivable for the Budget Year Ending December 31, 19x6

(thousands of dollars)

Month	Net Rev.	Due from ABC/HMO 0.05	Due from Pat. A/R	January	February	March	April	May	June	July	August	September	October	November	December	Total Cash Coll.	Uncoll. A/Rs
Monthly collection patterns				1st Mo. 0.333	2nd Mo. 0.269	3rd Mo. 0.187	4th Mo. 0.112	5th Mo. 0.04	6th Mo. 0.009								
Beg. Bal.	$ 1,500			$500	$404	$280	$168	$120	$ 28							$ 1,500	
January	856	$ 43	$ 813	285	230	160	95	34	9							813	
February	850	44	806		283	229	159	95	33	7						806	
March	832	43	789			277	224	155	93	33	7					789	
April	880	46	834				293	236	165	98	34	8				834	
May	787	45	742					262	212	142	88	31	7			742	
June	880	46	834						293	236	165	98	34	8		834	
July	850	44	806							283	228	159	95	34	7	806	
August	880	46	834								293	236	165	98	35	827	7
September	850	44	806									283	228	159	95	765	41
October	880	46	834										293	236	165	694	140
November	880	46	834											293	236	529	305
December	855	47	808												284	284	524
Subtotal	$10,280		$9,740	$785	$917	$946	$939	$902	$833	$799	$815	$815	$822	$828	$822	$10,223	$1,017
ABC/HMO		$540	540	43	44	43	46	45	46	44	46	44	46	46	47	540	
Net Rev.	$10,280		$10,280	$828	$961	$989	$985	$947	$879	$843	$861	$859	$868	$874	$869	$10,763	$1,017

Table 10-10 Analysis of Other Operating Cash Inflows for the Budget Year Ending
December 31, 19x6

			(thousands of dollars)			
Month	Rentals	Vending Machines	Medical Records	Cafeteria Sales	Gifts & Donations	Total
1	$ 15	$ 3	$ 2	$ 9	$10	$ 39
2	15	2	1	9	5	32
3	12	2	1	9	5	29
4	10	1	1	8	5	25
5	10	1	1	8	5	25
6	10	1	1	8	0	20
7	10	1	1	9	0	21
8	10	1	2	8	0	21
9	10	1	1	8	0	20
10	10	1	1	9	5	26
11	10	1	1	8	0	20
12	10	1	1	9	0	21
Total	$132	$16	$14	$102	$35	$299

Variable operating expenses comprise all the remaining expenses of the institution that tend to vary in proportion to the volume of activity and that are due and payable from the institution's account for trade payables. This type of expense can

Table 10-11 Cash Outflow Analysis of Salaries, Wages, and Related Expenses for the
Budget Year Ending December 31, 19x6

		(thousands of dollars)		
Month	Payroll Dates	Gross Monthly Payroll	Related Expenses	Total Expenses
1	10/1, 10/15	$ 320	$ 50	$ 370
2	11/1, 11/15	330	55	385
3	12/1, 12/15	340	60	400
4	1/1, 1/15	345	62	407
5	2/1, 2/15	345	62	407
6	3/1, 3/15	350	65	415
7	4/1, 4/15	350	65	415
8	5/1, 5/15	360	67	427
9	6/1, 6/15	360	67	427
10	7/1, 7/15	365	70	435
11	8/1, 8/15	365	70	435
12	9/1, 9/15	370	72	442
Total		$4,200	$765	$4,965

Table 10-12 Summary of Programmed Expenses for the Budget Year Ending December 31, 19x6

Month	Mortgage Payments	Leases & Rentals	Insurance	Utilities	Total
		(thousands of dollars)			
1	$ 150	$ 25	$ 40	$ 30	$ 245
2	150	25	—	30	205
3	150	25	—	30	205
4	150	25	40	30	245
5	150	25	—	30	205
6	150	25	—	30	205
7	150	25	40	30	245
8	150	25	—	30	205
9	150	25	—	30	205
10	150	25	45	30	250
11	150	25	—	30	205
12	150	25	—	30	205
Total	$1,800	$300	$165	$360	$2,625

and should be analyzed with the same method used to analyze accounts receivable (see Table 10-14). Priorities of payment (see Table 10-15) can assist management and the accounting department in paying the institution's accounts payable in a timely and orderly fashion.

Table 10-13 Schedule of Capital Expenditures for the Budget Year Ending December 31, 19x6

Month	Amount Required (in thousands)
1	$ 75
2	100
3	250
4	0
5	0
6	500
7	0
8	100
9	100
10	250
11	0
12	0
Total	$1,375

Table 10–14 Spreadsheet Analysis of Variable Accounts Payable and Payment Schedule for the Budget Year Ending December 31, 19x6

(thousands of dollars)

Month	Accounts Payable	1st Mo. 0.55	2nd Mo. 0.2	3rd Mo. 0.1	4th Mo. 0.15									Payment Total	Payables Balance
		1	2	3	4	5	6	7	8	9	10	11	12		
Beg. Bal.	130	72	26	13	19									130	0
1	148	81	30	15	22									148	0
2	134		74	27	13	20								134	0
3	142			78	28	14	22							142	0
4	170				93	34	17	26						170	0
5	158					87	32	16	23					158	0
6	152						84	30	15	23				152	0
7	158							87	31	16	24			158	0
8	160								88	32	16	24		160	0
9	158									87	31	16	24	158	0
10	162										89	33	16	138	24
11	164											90	34	124	40
12	164												90	90	74
Total	2000	153	130	133	175	155	155	159	157	158	160	163	164	1862	138

Table 10-15 Schedule of Payment Priorities for Accounts Payable for the Budget Year Ending December 31, 19x6

Priority Category	Type of Payment	Description of Payment	Payment Schedule from Date of Receipt
A	Programmed/fixed	Payroll, commissions, and other personnel related expenses	Current month
B	Programmed/fixed	Mortgage, rent, leases, rentals, utilities, loan payments, and service contracts	Current month
C	Variable	Food stuffs, medical & surgical, pharmaceuticals	Within 30 days (following month)
D	Variable	Accounts with trade and sales discounts	Within 30 days (following month)
E	Programmed/fixed	Funded depreciation	Within 30 days (following month)
F	Variable	Special vendors	30–59 days (second month)
G	Variable	Other vendors	60–90 days (third month)

MASTER CASH FLOW FORECAST

The master cash flow forecast (see Table 10-1) schedules the cash inflows and cash outflows as developed in the preceding tables. Line item 2E, borrowings (investments and/or payback), has been used as a balancing account. For example, the total cash outflow for month 1 was $893,000 but the cash-on-hand before the addition of $15,000 was only $882,000, an $11,000 shortfall. Consequently, $15,000 was added from borrowings. On the other hand, month 2 projected cash-on-hand of $998,000, which is $128,000 more than needed to meet the cash outflow of $870,000. Therefore, $115,000 was provided for payback on the previous month's borrowing and the balance was invested. What is important in this model is that each month's ending balance was maintained at a "reasonable" minimum: Excess cash was invested.

The total column of the cash flow statement summarizes all of the activities for the year, beginning with $10,000 in month 1 and ending with a $15,000 balance for month 12.

The master cash flow forecast can serve as the base from which to update the cash projection. The statement has been programmed on a microcomputer spreadsheet, and when the current totals have been entered, the system will automatically update itself and make adjustments for the remainder of the year. A health care institution's cash position is so vitally critical that it must be monitored every day. Exhibit 10-1 is an example of a daily cash report which has been designed from the original cash flow forecast.

Cash forecasting is undoubtedly one of the most important functions in health care financial management. If properly prepared and used, the cash forecast can help management to keep the organization financially viable by predicting cash shortfalls and excesses. With this knowledge, management can make timely and appropriate corrective decisions.

In summary, even though the institution's patient account manager has the ultimate responsibility for converting the organization's largest single asset—patient accounts receivable—to cash, all department managers, whether their department(s) generate revenue or not, must know the cash impact each has upon the institution's total cash flow. Cash management requires a total team effort to ensure the organization a steady and adequate cash flow.[7]

Exhibit 10-1 Daily Cash Report

Hometown Memorial Hospital
Hometown, U.S.A.

Daily Cash Report

as of _____ 19__

	Today	*Actual*	*Budget*	*Variance*
		MONTH-TO-DATE		
1. Beginning cash balance	$_____	$_____	$_____	$_____
2. Cash inflows				
A. Patient receivables	$_____	$_____	$_____	$_____
B. Negotiated contracts	_____	_____	_____	_____
C. Other operating sources	_____	_____	_____	_____
D. Investment income	_____	_____	_____	_____
E. Borrowings (investments)	_____	_____	_____	_____
F. Total cash inflows	$_____	$_____	$_____	$_____
3. Total cash-on-hand	$_____	$_____	$_____	$_____
4. Cash outflows				
A. Salaries, wages, etc.	$_____	$_____	$_____	$_____
B. Programmed expenses	_____	_____	_____	_____
C. Variable operating expenses	_____	_____	_____	_____
D. Funded depreciation	_____	_____	_____	_____
E. Capital expenditures	_____	_____	_____	_____
F. Other investments	_____	_____	_____	_____
G. Total cash outflows	$_____	$_____	$_____	$_____
5. Ending cash balance	$_____	$_____	$_____	$_____

NOTES

1. Corine T. Norgaard, *Management Accounting* (Englewood Cliffs, N.J.: Prentice-Hall, 1985), 253.
2. Ibid.
3. Allen G. Herkimer, Jr., *Understanding Hospital Financial Management*, 2d ed. (Rockville, Md.: Aspen, 1986), 303.
4. Ibid.
5. Ibid., 305.
6. Ibid., 306.
7. Ibid., 323.

Master Budget, Control Budget, and Variance Analysis

11

The process of developing departmental budgets with the involvement both of department managers and of administration might well also constitute the best management development program. This process forces all participants and their subordinates to examine thoroughly their own departments and responsibility centers; to identify formally the mission, goals, and objectives; to examine the marketplace and select the needs the institution can best serve; and to develop strategies designed to achieve the goals and objectives. After the planning process has been articulated, the budget serves as the financial instrument that expresses the narration in quantitative terms. The master budget, the product of the management team's best conceived strategy for the organization's future, cannot become a working document without the approval of the governing board. Therefore, the master budget must be packaged and organized so as to be (1) easily read and understood by individuals who may be interested only in the ''bottom line'' and (2) sufficiently amplified for those who want detail.

The master budget package must be brief and to the point so that the average individual can quickly understand both the narrative and the financial goals and objectives of the institution and its departments. For this reason, the packaging and presentation (to the board and department managers) of the budget must be given considerable time and thought: It is a product which needs to be sold.

PACKAGING THE BUDGET

There is no single correct method to use when preparing the budget for formal presentation. The method varies from one institution to another, from one management team to another. The development and packaging of a budget is like the creation of a fine sculpture: Both have been chiselled out of raw material and both need to be appraised, refined, reappraised, and refined again. The health care institution's management team must never be totally satisfied with the ''final'' budget. It must use each budget development process to fine tune both the process, the presentation, and the end result.

Following is a list of suggested contents for a budget package:

- executive summary
- table of contents
- list of illustrations and graphs (optional but *very* helpful)
- comparative income and expense summary (including volume of activity)
- unit value (Patient Day) analysis (optional but *very* helpful)
- budget balancers, if necessary
- mission, goals and objectives
- assumptions
- summary of departmental capital expenditures
- monthly departmental volume forecast summary
- monthly departmental revenue budget summary
- monthly departmental expense budget summary
- monthly cash flow forecast
- appendix

The executive summary can be likened to a newspaper's headlines. It can highlight all of the pertinent information for the reader who doesn't have the time or want to take the time to read a long detailed document or it can entice the reader to delve into the inner workings of the budget and its projected results. It's called an *executive summary*, and that's what it is—crisp, concise, and straight to the point for the busy executive.

A budget package is presented best when

- *all* of the master budget's pages are sorted according to subject and sequentially numbered
- a table of contents is placed at the beginning of the document
- all of the exhibits, graphs, and other supporting illustrations are sequentially numbered and cataloged in a list of illustrations

These are only a few of the checklist items for a well-packaged master budget; there may be many more topics and issues which management wants to have included in the master budget package so as to help the reviewer better understand it. The master budget packaging is a direct reflection on the character and professionalism of the individual who coordinated the budget process. A well-organized master budget helps to develop and enhance the credibility of the budget and the budget officer.

The comparative income and expense summary—or profit and loss (P&L) statement as it is sometimes called—is a financial statement which summarizes the institution's primary sources of income, its related application of expenses, and the net operating result (profit or loss). The statement offers to the reviewer an opportunity to compare the projected budget totals with those for other time periods, e.g., the previous year's actual totals, the current year's actual totals, the current budget year totals, etc. A suggested model for a comparative income and expense summary is displayed in Exhibit 11-1. This same format model can be used to develop a value unit (patient day) comparative analysis, illustrated in Table 11-1.

Exhibit 11-1 Comparative Income and Expense Summary

Hometown Memorial Hospital
Hometown, U.S.A.

Comparative Income and Expense Summary
for the Budget Year Ending December 31, 19x6

Description	Previous Year Actual	Current Year Actual	Proposed Budget
Volume			
Patient days			
Outpatient visits			
Operating Revenue			
Gross patient revenue	$_____	$_____	$_____
Less deductibles			
Net patient revenue	$_____	$_____	$_____
Operating Expenses			
Salaries and benefits	$_____	$_____	$_____
Nonsalary expenses			
Depreciation			
Total operating expenses	$_____	$_____	$_____
Net operating profit (loss)	$_____	$_____	$_____
Nonoperating revenue	$_____	$_____	$_____
Nonoperating expenses			
Net Nonoperating profit (loss)	$_____	$_____	$_____
Net profit (loss)	$_____	$_____	$_____

Table 11-1 Comparative Analysis of Selected Departmental Revenues and Expenses per Patient Day for the Budget Year Ending December 31, 19x6

Description	Previous Year Actual	Current Year Actual	Budget
Laboratory revenue	$ 12.75	$ 13.28	$ 12.98
Radiology expenses	$ 24.62	$ 25.89	$ 26.15
Housekeeping expenses	$ 3.41	$ 4.56	$ 4.87
I.C.U. revenue	$275.00	$289.00	$295.00
Medical & surgical nursing expenses	$156.89	$172.99	$185.42

Similar comparative studies help the reviewers to relate to an individual price or cost of service. It eliminates substantial dollar totals and differences because of volume fluctuations.

The budget must be compared to the actual totals of the previous and current years and not to the previous year's budget: Actual results are more meaningful than projections. This type of summary statement offers the reader a point of reference insofar as patient volume is concerned; the dollar value may change from year to year but patient days and visits remain relatively constant. Finally, it is imperative that operating revenues and expenses be separated from nonoperating revenues and expenses such as investment income, etc. This approach gives the reviewer(s) an opportunity to evaluate the results of operations apart from any subsidies from nonoperational activities.

If the revenue and expense summary statement includes the budget balancers, there is no need to include these in a separate section of the master budget. Budget balancers may be defined as individual revenue and/or expense adjustments to the preliminary budget which may be included so as to enable the final master budget to generate management's desired results. It is not necessary to identify any budget balancers if the revenue and expense summary statement is presented as a final budget. However, if management wants to initially display the preliminary budget summary statement and then highlight the major adjustments as budget balancers, it is essential to include these adjustments in a separate section of the master budget.

The institution's mission, goals, and objectives should also be consolidated, formalized, and incorporated into the master budget so that the reader has another point of reference for evaluating it.

One of the most trying and embarrassing experiences during the presentation of a budget to the governing board or to any other body of individuals can occur when the presenter is asked, for example, "What percentage did you use for the inflation rate?" or "How many hours of nursing care are budgeted for the I.C.U., the medical and surgical unit, and the pediatric unit?" Unless the presenter has a photographic memory or an unusual ability to recall details, such questions can cause frustration and possible embarrassment. It is advisable, therefore, to list the principle assumptions used to generate the budgeted results. These will provide the reviewer with most of the answers to typical questions before the meeting and will reduce the number of questions during the presentation.

A departmental summary or listing of the budgeted capital expenses is sufficient for most governing boards. However, it may be advisable to incorporate a monthly acquisition schedule in the master budget's appendix as supporting data to the listing.

When thinking about a budget, one usually visualizes long columns of dollar figures. Many people get completely lost in such a maze of data, so they immediately jump to the bottom line and investigate no further. Most people, especially board members, are keenly aware of dollar fluctuations from one year to another and find it difficult to compare the totals. For this reason, the monthly departmental volume forecast summary is critical. The statistics used in most budgetary programs (e.g., patient days, outpatient visits, etc.) are universally accepted and do not fluctuate in value from year to year. These types of statistics can serve as a good point of reference for the reviewer. The budget's statistical summary is usually enough for most reviewers; a detailed statistical analysis may be placed in the appendix of the master budget as supporting documentation.

The body of the institution's master budget usually includes only the monthly departmental revenue and expense summaries. If additional detail is required, it may be included in the master budget's appendix. It is important that the body of the master budget be easy for the reviewers to read. Only financial and statistical summaries should be incorporated in the body of the budget, while detailed worksheets (if required) may be placed in the appendix.

The monthly cash flow forecast is usually placed near the end of the body of the master budget. During the course of budget review, some major changes in revenues and expenses might be recommended, thus altering the projections of the cash flow forecast.

In summary, a few rules to keep in mind during the packaging process for the master budget are as follows:

- Make it simple, concise, and not wordy; most of all, use a reasonable amount of white space to facilitate reading.

- Highlight the important items and trends, but don't conceal anything or mislead the reviewers.

- Include in the body of the master budget only summaries and other supporting illustrations or graphs.

- Include in the appendix all required detailed worksheets, etc.

- Don't make the final master budget so bulky as to discourage its reading and use by the institution's board, the department managers, and the management team.

CONTROL BUDGET

The control budget may be defined as the basis of the performance evaluation process. It utilizes standard variable rates to adjust the target budget to the actual volume of activity, thus eliminating the necessity for rationalizing the dollar differences due to volume variances. The target budget is the fixed budget from which standard variable rates are generated. These standard rates, when multiplied by the actual volume of activity, provide the adjusted total variable expenses; the total fixed expenses of the target budget remain constant. The following methodology is designed for the development of a variable control budget:

1. Categorize all of the accounts in the health care institution's chart of accounts as either (1) salary or (2) nonsalary expenses.
2. Identify all the fixed expenses of these categories for each department (note: like expenses may be classified differently by each participating department).
3. Assume that all the remaining accounts are variable expenses.
4. Select the production unit which best measures and represents the volume of activity generated by each department. The unit *patient day* is frequently used to adjust the entire hospital's volume of activity.
5. Calculate the standard variable expense (or revenue) rate by dividing the target budget's projected volume of activity into the projected annual dollar expense (or revenue) of each departmental variable expense (or revenue) item.
6. Group the variable salary and nonsalary expense items separately at the top of the control budget.
7. Group the fixed salary and nonsalary expense items separately in the bottom section of the control budget; these amounts remain as listed in the target budget.
8. Provide a column next to the account description for the standard variable rate; compute the adjusted total variable expense for each item by multiplying the standard variable rates by the actual volume of activity.
9. Add all the subtotals of the four expense categories to arrive at the adjusted control budget total.

The budget in Table 11-2 is a fixed or target budget with a projected volume of 25,000 production units (visits) evaluated to an actual performance which gener-

Table 11-2 Emergency Services Department Comparative Analysis of Fixed Target Budget to Actual Performance for the Fiscal Year Ending September 30, 19x2

Description	Actual	Fixed Budget	Favorable (Unfavorable) Variance
Volume			
ER visits	23,500	25,000	(1,500)
Salary & Wage Expenses			
Management and supervision	$ 70,000	$ 68,000	$(2,000)
Physicians	190,000	185,000	(5,000)
Registered nurses	95,000	100,000	5,000
E.R. technicans	115,000	115,000	0
Admitting and clerical	90,000	91,000	1,000
Total salary & wage expenses	$560,000	$559,000	$(1,000)
Nonsalary Expenses			
Medical and surgical supplies	$123,000	$120,000	$(3,000)
Dues and subscriptions	10,000	12,000	2,000
Depreciation	70,000	70,000	0
Office supplies	24,000	25,000	1,000
Telephone	6,000	6,000	0
Equipment rentals	12,000	13,000	1,000
Total nonsalary expenses	$245,000	$246,000	$ 1,000
Total expenses	$805,000	$805,000	$ 0

ated 23,500 production units. According to this analysis, there is no financial variance between the total actual performance ($805,000) and the total targeted expenses ($805,000). A reviewer's initial reaction might be that this is a very favorable report.

At this point, no reference has been made to the volume of activity. The target budget was based on a volume of 25,000 visits, but there were only 23,500 actual visits. Using the standard variable expense rates developed in Table 11-3, the variable control budget in Table 11-4 demonstrates the significant differences in the performance reports based on a fixed and a variable budget.

Using the fixed budget methodology (see Table 11-2), no financial difference is identified between the actual performance and the budgeted total. The analysis does, however, identify the 1,500 fewer visits as an unfavorable variance between the volumes of activity. On the other hand, the variable control budget approach (see Table 11-4) identifies an unfavorable variance of $32,820. The cause of this total variance is reviewed in the following section.

Table 11-3 Computation of Target Budget Standard Variable Expense Rates for the Budget Year Ending September 30, 19x2

Projected Volume of Activity: 25,000 visits
Formula: column B/25,000 = column C

(A) Description	(B) Annual Total Expenses	(C) Standard Rate per Visit
Variable Expenses		
Salaries and wages		
Physicians	$185,000	$7.40
Registered nurses	100,000	4.00
ER technicians	115,000	4.60
Nonsalary		
Medical & surgical supplies	$123,000	$4.92
Office supplies	24,000	.96

Table 11-5 is a comparative analysis of the results of the fixed and variable control budget approaches. The difference is that the variable control approach eliminates the necessity for rationalizing the differences caused by volume variances.

PERFORMANCE ANALYSIS

The objective of performance analysis is to recognize potential problems which may be developing and to take timely corrective actions as opportunities present themselves. The cost control model shown in Figure 11-1 identifies the major stages in any situation requiring cost control within an organization.[1] The three distinct stages are as follows:

1. the recognition of the problem (t_0 to t_1)
2. the determination of the problem cause (t_1 to t_2)
3. the correction of the problem (t_2 to t_3)

The model's unit of time may be minutes, hours, days, weeks, or even months. The important point is that the longer the problem remains uncorrected (t_0 to t_3), the greater the cost to the health care institution.

Efficiency cost is the term which is sometimes used to identify the total cost incurred by an organization from an out-of-control cost situation. Efficiency cost may be computed using the following formula:

Table 11-4 Emergency Services Department Comparative Analysis of Variable Control Budget to Actual Performance for the Fiscal Year Ending September 30, 19x2

Description	Standard Rate	Control Budget	Actual	Favorable (Unfavorable) Variance
Volume				
ER visits		23,500	23,500	0
Variable Expenses				
Salary and wages				
Physicians	$7.40	$173,900	$190,000	$(17,000)
Registered nurses	4.00	94,000	95,000	(1,000)
E.R. technicians	4.60	108,100	115,000	(6,900)
Total variable salary & wages		$376,000	$400,000	$(24,000)
Nonsalary				
Med & surg supplies	$4.92	$115,620	$123,000	$ (7,380)
Office supplies	.96	22,560	24,000	(1,440)
Total nonsalary variable expenses		$138,180	$147,000	$ (8,820)
Total variable expenses		$514,180	$547,000	$(32,820)
Fixed Expenses				
Salary & wages				
Management & supervision		$ 68,000	70,000	$ (2,000)
Clerical		91,000	90,000	1,000
Total fixed salary & wages		$159,000	160,000	$ (1,000)
Nonsalary				
Dues and subscriptions		$ 12,000	$ 10,000	$ 2,000
Depreciation		70,000	70,000	0
Telephone		6,000	6,000	0
Rentals		13,000	12,000	1,000
Total fixed nonsalary expenses		$101,000	$ 98,000	$ 3,000
Total fixed expenses		$260,000	$258,000	$ 2,000
Total fixed & variable expenses		$774,180	$805,000	$(34,820)

$$\text{Efficiency cost} = T \times R \times P$$

where

T = total time units that the problem remains uncorrected

R = loss (or cost) per time unit

P = probability that the problem occurrence is correctable

The object of performance analysis is to identify cost variances to the budget and to minimize the efficiency cost in any given situation.[2] For the purpose of this study, performance analysis has been divided into two major expense categories:

Table 11-5 Emergency Services Department Comparative Analysis of the Fixed and Variable Control Budget Approaches for the Budget Year Ending September 30, 19x2

Description	Actual Performance	Target Budget	Control Budget
Volume			
ER visits	23,500	25,000	23,500
Variable Expenses			
Salary & wages	$400,000	$400,000	$376,000
Nonsalary	147,000	145,000	138,180
Total variable expenses	$547,000	$545,000	$514,180
Fixed Expenses			
Salary & wages	$160,000	$159,000	$159,000
Nonsalary	98,000	101,000	101,000
Total fixed expenses	$258,000	$260,000	$260,000
Total Fixed & Variable Expenses	$805,000	$805,000	$774,180

1. salary and wages

   - rate variance
   - efficiency variance

2. nonsalary

   - rate variance
   - usage variance

The rate variance identifies the difference between the target budget (standard) rate and the actual cost and multiplies this amount by the actual volume of activity to compute the total rate variance per expense item.

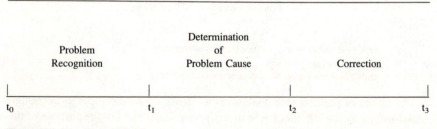

Figure 11-1 Cost Control Model

The efficiency and usage variances are similar in that they recognize differences in the amount of resources (e.g., person-hours or production units) and multiply these differences by the target budget (standard) cost to determine the total variance cost for each expense account.

Inefficiency costs are minimized when the problem or opportunity is recognized quickly. For this reason, it is imperative that *each* expense account be analyzed for performance variances, as illustrated in the analyses in Tables 11-6 and 11-7.

As illustrated in Table 11-6, the emergency services department experienced a $6,570 favorable salary and wage efficiency variance, computed as follows:

	Hours		*Fav(Unfav)*	*Budget*	*Efficiency*
Position	*Target*	*Actual*	*Variance*	*Rate*	*Variance*
Physicians	6,167	6,129	38	$30.00	$1,140
Registered nurses	6,667	6,552	115	15.00	1,725
ER technicians	15,333	14,839	494	7.50	3,705
Total	28,167	27,520	647		$6,570

Each position experienced a favorable variance (totaling 647 hours) by using fewer hours than budgeted. Computing these variances by the positions' budgeted hourly rates results in an accumulated total of $6,570 in efficiency variances.

On the other hand, the department realized an unfavorable salary and wage rate variance totaling $6,562.75, computed as follows:

	Hourly Rate		*Fav(Unfav)*	*Hours*	*Rate*
Position	*Target*	*Actual*	*Variance*	*Worked*	*Variance*
Physicians	$30.00	$31.00	$(1.00)	6,129	$(6,129.00)
Registered nurses	15.00	14.50	.50	6,552	3,276.00
ER technicians	7.50	7.75	(.25)	14,839	(3,709.75)
Total				27,520	$(6,562.75)

Both the physicians and the ER technicians had a greater hourly rate than had been budgeted, thus accumulating a total of $9,838.75 unfavorable rate variance. This was partially offset by a $3,276.00 favorable rate variance (with respect to registered nurses), thus netting out to a total unfavorable rate variance of $6,562.75.

The validity of these analyses is verified by adding the total salary and wage expense variances in the "proof" summary in Table 11-6 and comparing this total to the difference as identified in Table 11-2:

Table 11-6 Emergency Services Department Performance Analysis of Variable Salary and Wage Expenses for the Budget Year Ending September 30, 19x2

Description	Physicians	Registered Nurses	Emergency Room Technicians	Total
1. Target budget standards				
A. Budget hourly rate	$30.00	$15.00	$7.50	
B. Budget hours	6,167	6,667	15,333	28,167
C. Target budget	$185,000	$100,000	$115,000	$400,000
(Lines 1A × 1B = 1C)				
2. Control budget standard				
A. Standard hourly rate	$30.00	$15.00	$7.50	
B. Actual hours worked	6,129	6,552	14,839	27,520
C. Control budget	$183,870	$98,280	$111,292	$393,442
(Lines 2A × 2B = 2C)				
3. Actual performance				
A. Actual hourly rate	$31.00	$14.50	$7.75	
B. Actual hours worked	6,129	6,552	14,839	27,520
C. Actual performance	$190,000	$95,000	$115,000	$400,000
(Lines 3A × 3B = 3C)				
4. Efficiency variance				
A. Target budget hours	6,167	6,667	15,333	28,167
B. Actual hours worked	6,129	6,552	14,839	27,520
C. Hour variance	38	115	494	647
D. Standard hourly rate	$30.00	$15.00	$7.50	
E. Efficiency variance	$1,140	$1,725	$3,705	$6,570
(Lines 4C × 4D = 4E)				
5. Rate variance				
A. Actual hours worked	6,129	6,552	14,839	27,520
B. Actual hourly rate	$31.00	$14.50	$7.75	
C. Standard hourly rate	$30.00	$15.00	$7.50	
D. Hourly rate variance	$1.00	($0.50)	$0.25	$0.75
E. Rate variance	$6,129.00	($3,276.00)	$3,709.75	$6,562.75
(Lines 5A × 5D = 5E)				
6. Total variances	$7,269.00	($1,551.00)	$7,414.75	$13,132.75
7. Proof				
A. Target budget	$185,000	$100,000	$115,000	$400,000
B. Actual performance	$190,000	$95,000	$115,000	$400,000
C. Variance target to actual	($5,000)	$5,000	$0	$0

Table 11-7 Emergency Services Department Variable Analysis of Variable Nonsalary Expenses for the Budget Year Ending September 30, 19x2

Description	Med & Surg Supplies	Office Supplies	Total
1. Usage variance			
A. Target budget volume	25,000	25,000	
B. Actual volume	23,500	23,500	
C. Volume variance	1,500	1,500	
D. Target budget unit rate	$ 4.80	$ 1.00	
E. Usage variance	$ 7,205.00	$ 1,500.00	$ 8,705
(Lines 1C × 1D = 1E)			favorable
2. Rate variance			
A. Target budget unit rate	$ 4.80	$ 1.00	
B. Actual unit cost	$ 5.23	$ 1.02	
C. Unit cost variance	$ 0.43	$ 0.02	
D. Actual volume	23,500	23,500	
E. Rate variance	$ 10,105.00	$ 470.00	$ (10,575)
(Lines 2C × 2D = 2E)			unfavorable
3. Total variances	$ 2,900.00	$1,030.00	$ (1,870)
			unfavorable
4. Proof			
A. Target budget	$ 120,000.00	$ 25,000.00	$ 145,000
B. Actual performance	$ 123,000.00	$ 24,000.00	$ 147,000
C. Total variance	$ (3,000.00)	$ 1,000.00	$ (2,000)
			unfavorable

Position	Target Budget	Actual Performance	Fav(Unfav) Variance
Physicians	$185,000	$190,000	$(5,000)
Registered nurses	100,000	95,000	5,000
ER technicians	115,000	115,000	0
Total	$400,000	$400,000	$ 0

The net difference of $7.25 results from rounding out the totals and the rates.

Similar types of variance analyses are done for the nonsalary expense portion of the financial statements as illustrated in Table 11-7.

The total favorable usage variance of $8,705 is composed of favorable variances of $7,205 for medical and surgical supplies and $1,500 for office supplies. These, however, are offset by the accumulated unfavorable rate or price variance of $10,575 (composed of $10,105 for medical and surgical supplies and $470 for office supplies). The net total of unfavorable nonsalary expense variances of

$1,870 (see Table 11-7) is a difference of $130 from the proof total variances of $2,000; again, this difference results from rounding out dollars.

To summarize, variances indicate which salary and wage positions were paid at rates different from those budgeted. For each position, the rate difference multiplied by the hours worked gives the total rate variance for the position. The efficiency variance determines (for each position) the difference between actual hours worked and the budgeted hours. The difference is then multiplied by the budgeted standard rate to compute the total variance. The usage variance identifies differences caused by using more or less of a nonsalary expense item because of volume changes. The volume variance is multiplied by the target budget standard cost per unit to arrive at the amount of the usage variance. The rate variance of nonsalary expenses is similar to the rate variance in analyzing salary and wage expenses. The difference between the actual unit cost and the target budget unit cost is calculated and multiplied by the actual volume of activity to compute the rate variance for each nonsalary expense item. These types of variance analyses, together with the variable control budget, help the reviewers to locate potential problems in either the budgeting process or operations.

PERFORMANCE REPORTS

There are as many formats for management reports as there are financial managers and department managers in the health care industry. Each performance report must be designed and created exclusively for the user and for the individual health care organization, but some general principles are as follows:[3]

- Reports should be tailored to organizational structure (responsibilities).
- Reports should be designed to implement the management exception principle, and they should include a basis for evaluation of performance.
- Reports should be simple and understandable.
- Reports should contain only essential information.
- Reports should be adapted to the needs and personal preferences of the primary users.
- Reports should be designed with particular consideration given to their primary use.
- Reports should be accurate.
- Reports should be prepared and presented promptly.
- Reports, when possible, should be constructive rather than critical in tone.
- Reports should be standardized where feasible.

One of the most important principles is to make the report easier to read by using proper spacing, especially minimizing the required "eye span" from a narrative description to the numerical data. The performance report in Exhibit 11-2 illustrates an appropriate format for such a report.

Performance reports which communicate effectively to all levels of management facilitate understanding, stimulate corrective action, and influence the decision-making process. (Note that graphs can contribute greatly to a report's effectiveness.) Those charged with the design and preparation of performance reports must know and understand the needs and methods of management.

Total management involvement and communication are the essential ingredients of an effective budgetary control program. Using a control budget elimi-

---

Exhibit 11-2 Sample Format for a Performance Report

Hometown Memorial Hospital
Hometown, U.S.A.

Emergency Services Department
Comparative Income and Expense Statement
for the Budget Year Ending September 30, 19x2

This Month				Year-to-Date		
Actual	*Budget*	*Variance*	*Description*	*Actual*	*Budget*	*Variance*
			Volume:			
____	____	____	Number of units	____	____	____
			Revenue:			
____	____	____	Gross patient revenue	____	____	____
____	____	____	Less deductions	____	____	____
____	____	____	Net patient revenue	____	____	____
			Expenses:			
____	____	____	Fixed salary & wages	____	____	____
____	____	____	Fixed nonsalary	____	____	____
____	____	____	Total fixed expense	____	____	____
____	____	____	Variable salary & wage	____	____	____
____	____	____	Variable nonsalary	____	____	____
____	____	____	Total variable expenses	____	____	____
____	____	____	Total expenses	____	____	____
____	____	____	Net profit (loss)	____	____	____

nates many questions about the differences due to variations in volumes of activity. The variance analysis procedures help management to identify differences due specifically to rates paid, usage of resources, and productivity of paid personnel.

NOTES

1. J. Stallman, "A Framework for Evaluating Cost Control Procedures for a Process," *Accounting Review* 4 (October 1972):774–87.

2. William O. Cleverly, *Handbook of Health Care Accounting and Finance* (Rockville, Md.: Aspen, 1982), 182–84.

3. Glenn A. Welsch, *Budgeting: Profit Planning and Control*, 2d ed. (Englewood Cliffs, N.J.: Prentice-Hall, 1964), 362.

Chapter 12

Humantology of Health Care Budgeting

12

The average health care organization has at its disposal as wide a spectrum of human resources as any other industry. From the dietary maids and the housekeeping janitors to the registered nurses and physicians, the employees of any health care institution constitute its most valuable asset. In addition, they are the key to a successful budgetary control program.

It has been stated that we can automate the mechanics of budgeting but we cannot automate the humantology of budgeting.[1]

The humantology of health care budgeting may be defined as the tempered and responsive application by management of the basic principles that employees should have trust placed in them and that they should be encouraged to participate appropriately in the budget process in order to achieve the established budgetary goals of a health care institution.[2] One of the principles of humantology—that people should be trusted to perform adequately—is based on the hypothesis that such trust will be substantiated by results.[3]

Many of the shortcomings attributed to budgets are due to poor interpersonnel relations and poor attitudes on the part of management. By and large, the human element is the dominant factor in effective budgetary management.[4]

Obviously, the budget and the budgeting process in itself can accomplish nothing. The individuals using it determine whether it is administered well or badly. Sound budgeting must be based on such fundamentals as recognition of accomplishment, consideration for the rights of individuals, and fair play—in other words, on enlightened behavior by people.[5]

To evaluate the degree of humantology in the budgeting process, the following elements must be considered:

- the degree of individual participation
- the amount of group cohesiveness
- the level of aspiration and achievement

INDIVIDUAL PARTICIPATION

The administration of the average health care institution has become so complex that no one individual can effectively manage the entire operation. Management and control of the daily activities is a team effort, with the department manager on the front line. The involvement of the department managers is absolutely necessary for the success of any project.

The real value of participation at all management levels, aside from better planning, results from the psychological benefits that occur: A high degree of participation is conducive to better morale and greater initiative.[6] However, there is such a thing as "pseudoparticipation," that is, participation which looks like, but is not, full-fledged participation.[7] When pseudoparticipation is present, the primary elements of humantology, faith and trust, are jeopardized. If department managers suspect that they are being overlooked or ignored, they will start believing that they are being manipulated and that management is "pulling the wool over their eyes." Credibility, integrity, and trust in the executive office are then at risk. Faith and trust depend on there being deep-seated confidence among all levels of management.

Participation is not a panacea. There is evidence that it is inappropriate in certain environments or circumstances. When participation is encouraged, the standard methods of control may need modification.[8]

In an industrial setting, a study was conducted to investigate the effects of participation on production after work changes were introduced. If employee turnover and stated grievances can be taken as a measure of morale, then it seems clear that the test group which participated in the initiation of changes was better disposed toward their job situations than were the no-participation group. Using this study alone, one cannot decide if participation directly increased the incentive to produce (as measured by subsequent productivity) or only improved morale (which in turn led to increased production). This is a point worth considering, since morale is not perfectly correlated with productivity. However, the study does suggest that morale and/or productivity are enhanced as a result of employee participation in the initiation of change.[9]

GROUP COHESIVENESS

Group cohesiveness is another benefit of encouraging participation in the development of the health care organization's budget. Group cohesiveness may be defined as attraction to the group, desire to become or remain a member, and reluctance to leave the group. Another way of understanding or measuring group cohesiveness is the amount of "we" feeling generated in an individual as a result of his or her association with others. One study indicates that highly cohesive groups more frequently accept induction (direction) than do groups with low cohesiveness. This study also suggests that with participation held constant (all groups working under constant conditions), change in productivity is related to cohesiveness. Cohesiveness appears to be directly related to morale.[10]

Since participation seems to affect both cohesiveness and productivity and cohesiveness without participation also seems to affect productivity, the most likely conclusion is that cohesiveness is dependent on participation but that changes in productivity are more directly related to cohesiveness.[11]

THE LEVEL OF ASPIRATION AND ACHIEVEMENT

Budget participation results in a plan of action that includes a projected set of desired results and an estimate of the cost required to achieve these results. If participation has been successful, then the proposed budget levels of cost and results are accepted as goals and objectives by the participants and the budgeted results become the standards or levels of aspiration for the department managers. In an efficiently managed health care organization, the department manager influences the acceptance of these standards by the department's employees.

A level of aspiration is a goal one explicitly undertakes to reach rather than a goal one hopes to achieve.[12] The degree of effort expended by the department managers as they attempt to achieve the organization's budgeted goals and objectives is partially dependent on the levels of aspiration.

In one study, the levels of aspiration of individuals of roughly equivalent ability were measured before their performance on a variety of mathematical problems; it was discovered that the subjects with higher initial levels of aspiration performed more successfully. Based on a study of this nature, one might conclude that greater motivation to succeed is associated with higher levels of aspiration. Given that increased motivation leads to increased effort, increased performance would usually be the result.[13]

BUDGET FEEDBACK

Individual participation, group cohesiveness, and high levels of aspiration will be useless without feedback. Budget feedback is a process of two-way communication (oral and written) among all of the participants in the budget preparation process. Budget feedback must be timely. The budgetary control office informs the department managers how well their performance matched the budget; the department managers inform the budgetary control office why they performed as they did.

Regardless of how well the participation program was developed and how high the level of aspiration, the responsible department manager will very soon lose enthusiasm if the budgetary control office fails to communicate the results of comparing the actual performance and the budget in a timely manner. Absence of feedback will not only adversely affect the department's productivity, but it will also affect the manager's departmental morale.[14]

In a study designed to determine the effects of feedback on communication, it was discovered that task accuracy increased as feedback increased. It was also found that "zero" feedback is accompanied by low confidence and hostility while "free" feedback is accompanied by high confidence and amity.[15]

The budget is not designed to reduce the managerial function to a formula. It is a managerial tool, one purpose of which is to measure subsequent performance against the budgetary plan.[16] The control function is the most important phase of the budgetary control process. The disclosure of the need for remedial action (feedback) and the taking of remedial (corrective) action are just as important as the original drafting of the budget. To be effective, the feedback and corrective action processes must be systematically organized and made integral functions of the budgetary control program.

HUMAN RELATIONS ASPECTS OF BUDGETING

In exploring budgeting principles as they relate to people, the first consideration should be the motivation for the budget system. Why have one at all? Is the budget merely that part of the system of overall planning which informs all concerned how much to spend and assures that actions will occur by design rather than by accident. Or is the budget a pressure device designed to goad people to greater effort? It takes a little soul-searching to determine honestly which of these views represents the position of management in a particular institution.[17]

Some guidelines for budgetary control programs are as follows:

- Seek the approval and active participation of top management, including the governing board.
- Ensure there is a well-designed organizational structure, with clear-cut lines of responsibility.
- Document each department manager's area of responsibility and lines of authority.
- Use an accounting and statistical reporting and recording system which is coordinated with the organizational structure and collects required data for internal control and for external surveillance.

- Do not allow the budget to be used as a weapon; it should be considered only as a planning document which establishes operating objectives and standards for evaluating performance.
- Differentiate between the staff responsibilities of the budget director and the line responsibilities of the department managers.

STAFF VERSUS LINE RESPONSIBILITIES

The budget director's enthusiasm for an effective budget program can become contagious and affect the whole institution, but sometimes this enthusiastic individual oversteps his or her area of responsibility and alienates the department managers. This is not always due to a wish for power; it can be due to a zealous determination to develop an effective and efficient budgetary control program. Staff personnel must not attempt, or give the impression of attempting, to usurp line authority. Misconceptions about the function of the budget director in his or her accounting and budgeting activities frequently create friction.[18]

Staff personnel must never be required to exercise authority over operating (line) personnel. The budget director should not develop the budget for the department manager; that is a line responsibility. Neither should the budget director discuss operating deficiencies with operating personnel; that, too, is a line responsibility of the department manager.

The primary duty of the budget director is to coordinate the budget development process and the collection, recording, and reporting of actual performance as compared with budgeted standards. Included is responsibility for the design and direction of the budgetary control program; not included is responsibility for enforcing the budget. It is important to make a clear distinction between enforcing the budget and reporting a comparison of actual results and budget objectives. The budget director is responsible for reporting to all levels of operating management the results of operations related to the budgeted plan. Corrective actions, resulting from either favorable or unfavorable results, are strictly line functions.

A secondary function of the budget director is to act as "financial advisor" to all levels of management, but this activity must be exercised with discretion.

The budget director should avoid being placed in the position of approving budgets or taking line action concerning efficient or inefficient operating results outside of his or her own department. The budget director is responsible only for the design, implementation, and coordination of an effective cost control system and not for actual cost control and cost reduction.[19] Direct responsibility for cost control and reduction belongs to the department managers. However, the department managers should be reminded not to concentrate on such short-term goals as "return on investment" or "budget profits" at the expense of the institution's long-term goals.

Finally, documented delineation between staff and line responsibilities is an absolute necessity for any effective budgetary control program.

BUDGET: A PEOPLE PROJECT

It has been observed that prospering nations are those whose economic systems unleash the full measure of their people's energy, ability, character, and initiative and allow them the freedom to make the most of their opportunities.[20]

One of the key words in this observation is *people*.

- People's energy
- People's ability
- People's character
- People's initiative

The other key word is *freedom*.

- Freedom to make and create
- Freedom to use one's abilities
- Freedom to demonstrate one's character
- Freedom to exploit one's initiative

Collectively, the people of any health care enterprise, when properly motivated and directed, constitute an invaluable resource of synergistic talent and energy. The budgetary control program is an excellent means of promoting and utilizing the latent forces within people.

A health care budget is a people project. The preliminary elements of any effective budget program demand these two key factors:

- **PEOPLE** to perform assigned tasks
- **FREEDOM** to efficiently and effectively complete them

There must also be complete cooperation and communication throughout the entire institution.

FUTURE USES OF BUDGETS

Health care budgeting and the types of information generated can be expanded and used for purposes other than the traditional internal planning and control processes. For example, they can play key roles in negotiating risk-based contracts, e.g., HMOs, PPOs, IPAs, CMPs, etc. The list of current and future risk-based contracts is and will continue to be endless.

The key factor in any of these types of contract negotiations is that the health care manager must know the costs of the negotiated services. Without this information the institution will be handicapped in its search for a working agreement with another entity and will continue to be throughout the negotiations. The other party knows approximately what it wants to pay for the services; if the health care organization is not sufficiently prepared and doesn't know what its cost are, it should not be at the negotiating table—the results might be economically and professionally disastrous. It is imperative, therefore, that the health care institution's budget be generated in such a way as to simulate the "what if" situations before and during the risk-based negotiating process.

One of this book's purposes is to introduce the concept of budgeting to a health care organization's department managers. These technicians, who must assume the additional responsibility of being departmental financial managers, must be totally familiar with cost behaviors and budgetary control devices. They must know how to calculate the costs of the services their departments generate. In addition, they must become familiar with the kinds of budget simulation which computer technology offers to the financial manager.

This book has been designed to encourage all health care managers to become acquainted not only with the concept of health care budgeting, but also with the versatility of the microcomputer spreadsheet applications. It is the author's hope that department managers will assume a greater role in institutional cost control, cost reduction, and cost avoidance programs. Financial planning and budgetary control require—in fact, demand—teamwork and the resulting synergism. It might be helpful in devising a successful budgetary control process to keep the following principles in mind:

- Budgeting is essentially a process which, when properly implemented, distributes varying degrees of responsibility among an organization's personnel, including staff employees.
- Budgeting produces documents which, when appropriately used, can enhance the morale of the entire organization and improve its financial viability.

Finally, the budgetary control process is never perfect—nor should it be. Rather, the budgeting process and its results should be constantly reviewed, adjusted, and refined with each iteration. Like sterling silver, which maintains its luster and sheen through routine use, budgeting requires continued and constant polishing through application.

The budget should be a living document within every health care institution.

NOTES

1. Allen G. Herkimer, Jr., *Concepts of Hospital Financial Management,* 2d ed. (San Marcos, Tex.: Alfa Management Services, 1973), 91–92.

2. Ibid., 91.

3. Ibid.

4. Glenn A. Welsch, *Budgeting: Profit Planning and Control,* 2d ed. (Englewood Cliffs, N.J.: Prentice-Hall, 1964), 459–60.

5. Ibid. 459.

6. B.H. Lord and Glenn A. Welsch, *Business Budgeting* (New York: Controllership Foundation, 1958), 97.

7. Chris Argyris, *The Impact of Budgets on People* (New York: Controllership Foundation, 1958), 28.

8. Selwyn Becker and David Green, Jr., "Budgeting and Employee Behavior," *Journal of Business,* October 1962; reprinted in *Readings in Cost Accounting, Budgeting and Control,* ed. William E. Thomas, Jr. (Cincinnati, Ohio: South Western Publishing, 1968).

9. Ibid., 59–61.

10. S. Schachter et al., "An Experimental Study of Cohesiveness and Productivity," *Human Relations* 4 (1951): 228–38.

11. Ibid.

12. Ibid.

13. Ibid.

14. Herkimer, *Concepts of Hospital Financial Management,* 99–101.

15. H.J. Leavitt and R.A.H. Mueller, "Some Effects of Feedback on Communications," *Human Relations* 4 (1951): 401–10.

16. Herkman C. Hesser, *Budgeting: Principles and Practice* (New York: Ronald Press, 1959), 48.

17. Welsch, *Budgeting,* 459.

18. Ibid., 460.

19. Ibid.

20. Herkimer, *Concepts of Hospital Financial Management,* 75–77.

Index

Note: Pages appearing in *italics* indicate entries found in artwork and tables.